Fourteen Years

How I Struggled

Through Failure

and Became a

Successful Mother

Neveen Musa

Fourteen Years
Copyright © 2020 by Neveen Musa.

All rights reserved. No part of this publication may be reproduced, distributed or transmitted in any form or by any means, including photocopying, recording, or other electronic or mechanical methods, without the prior written permission of the publisher, except in the case of brief quotations embodied in critical reviews and certain other noncommercial uses permitted by copyright law.

Cover Design by 100Covers.com
Interior Design by FormattedBooks.com

ISBN: 978-1-7354220-0-8 (Paperback)

To everyone who is suffering silently,

trying hard to reach their dream,

and

is tired of failure.

You will get there. I believe in you.

Contents

SECTION 1: MY STORY 1

Introduction 3
Chapter 1: New Beginnings 5
Chapter 2: Marriage and Hope 9
Chapter 3: Going Home 16
Chapter 4: Back to Square One 22
Chapter 5: Our Next Move? 27
Chapter 6: Another Chance 32
Chapter 7: A Shift in Thinking 37
Chapter 8: Taking Responsibility 40
Chapter 9: Self-Reflection 45
Chapter 10: Continuing My Journey 48
Chapter 11: Staying Strong 53
Chapter 12: Being Fearless 60
Chapter 13: Getting Ready 64
Chapter 14: The Big Day 68
Chapter 15: Survival 73

SECTION 2: PERSONAL GROWTH 79

Introduction 81
Chapter 16: Time Management and Organization 83
Chapter 17: Persevere and Have Patience 89
Chapter 18: Acceptance and Change 94
Chapter 19: Failure and Forgiveness 98
Chapter 20: Believe and Have Faith 101
Chapter 21: Reward and Appreciation 105
Chapter 22: Expectations and Reasons 109
Chapter 23: Find Happiness 113

Final Thoughts 115

Section One

MY STORY

Introduction

My name is Neveen Musa. I am a wife, daughter, elementary school educator, fertility warrior, author, and now, a Mother. That is my favorite title of all. I've always followed my passion in life to reach my dreams. Whether it was being a teacher, businesswoman, motivator, or life changer, I have worked hard to achieve my goals.

For most of my life, I was living like most people, dealing with problems and issues as they arrived. I sought help though motivational programs to learn self-development skills, but nothing seemed to really change me or solve my life problems. Happiness was very hard to achieve sometimes because my life was full of problems, and I didn't have the life skills to deal with them.

Infertility became the biggest obstacle that my husband and I would strive to overcome so far.

Stress was my companion for over a decade. I became depressed and suffered in silence. Disappointment and heartache became the norm. I pictured myself coming to the end of the road of life and realizing that I had given up on my dreams. It took me waking up and accepting that I needed to change my mindset, my life, and start reaching for my dreams again.

I promised myself that when I achieved my goals, I would write a book to help others and to spread hope. Join me as I talk about my difficult journey with infertility. Throughout this book, I will explain the steps and stages of life that I went through and how I applied the skills and tools I learned along the way to reach my own dream of becoming a mother. I hope that my story can inspire others to dream and find their own kind of happiness.

In this book, I first take you through our infertility journey. After you read my story, I focus on some of the key aspects of my progress and break each one down to show you how you can reach your own goals too.

Chapter 1

New Beginnings

On a rainy day in December, the smell of burnt wood filled the air of our small village. I wore my light pink maxi dress and matched it with a soft beige hijab. I applied soft makeup to keep the look chic and natural. Today was a special day. Ali, my husband-to-be, had come with his family to visit my family as part of a traditional process before marriage. He was wearing a navy sweater with black pants and a leather jacket to complete his classy look.

My parents' house is located on a hill with the village in front of it. The view that day was breathtaking as the soft fall of rain added its romance to the fields. The smell of roasted Arabic coffee and a subtle lavender candle filled the house. Both sets of parents were sitting in the family room, and I waited for my father to call me to join them. I finally greeted everyone and sat next to my father. He permitted Ali and I to sit in the living room together alone to have a conversation and decide if we wanted to keep going with our courtship and get to know each other better.

In other words, this was like a first date for us.

It was my first time seeing Ali and talking to him alone. I felt a mixture of emotions, both shyness and nervousness. In my small village in Palestine, the heart of the Middle East, people know each other. They are all related in various ways: cousins, in-laws, family, neighbors, and friends.

Turmusaya, my village, is set between mountains and green plains. Olive trees, fig trees, grapes, and citrus trees fill the gardens. Each house is unique in its design and has its own huge garden around it. In winter, it can get pretty cold, and to keep the houses warm, almost every house has a fireplace. This fills the air of the village with that burning wood smell that I love. In Turmussaya, most of the village residents are American citizens. They go back and forth between the United States and the village. Almost every house is missing one family member because they traveled to the U.S. seeking a better life and future.

In our culture, before a couple can start to get to know each other, the future groom should come and ask the parents of the potential bride for permission to court her. This period is called engagement and ours lasted for seven months. Ali and I were a perfect match! We agreed on a lot of things, but disagreed on more issues. It is kind of a weird relationship. I think that people would say we "complete each other." We do have a lot of disagreements, but I just call it having a different point of view. We both respected each other's opinion. Seven months were enough time to decide to take the next step and get married.

On a lovely summer day in July, Ali and I began our traditional three-day wedding celebration. I was nineteen, and he was twenty-five. The first day of the celebration is the preparation for the wedding in which families gather at the groom's house to dance and sing while women prepare henna. I wore a traditional Palestinian dress called a *thob* that has uniquely handmade stitches with very colorful patterns.

The second day was the women's party when women gathered in one of the village banquet halls to dance and celebrate. I wore a very big and fluffy lavender dress like Cinderella might have worn. That was my taste back then, which was trendy at the time. On that night, men gathered to dance and perform a traditional dance called the *Dabka*. They celebrated until midnight, eating sweets, and ended the party with a light dinner.

The third day was the wedding. It was finally the big day! I was in the hair salon by 8:00 a.m. to have my hair and makeup done. I loved the way I looked, and Ali's reaction when he picked me up was priceless. I wore a rented, fancy white dress with handmade sequins and embroidery. I had a long matching veil and hair accessories to complete the look. I applied soft perfume, and overall, I looked like a princess. I felt like a princess, too.

Everyone in the village gathered and came to my parents' house to take me from my family home with singing and celebration. In the middle of the day, all of the villages were invited for dinner, which took place in a huge banquet hall. We spent the rest of that day celebrating together, sharing our first dance, cutting a cake, and taking pictures.

In my beautiful white wedding dress and with Ali in his handsome black tuxedo, we said our vows and started our new life. We supported each other as much as we could in our new marriage. We were moving to the United States a couple of weeks after our wedding day, and though we both had some fear, we knew we were seeking a better life and future. In August, we headed to the United States of America to begin our new life in a new country. Thankfully, we had extended family in Chicago, and they supported us and helped us acclimate to all the changes that our move brought.

Ever since we were married, I wanted to be a mother. Actually, it was something that I wanted to be since I was very young. We even discussed names for our future children while we were engaged. I had always loved children and babies. Aren't they the most incredible human beings, "When I felt depressed, just looking at their smiles made me forget my troubles and stress." We both wanted to have children and start a family right away.

I was suffering from an irregular menstrual cycle and the doctor diagnosed me with polycystic ovary syndrome (PCOS), which is fairly common. It was odd because I wasn't overweight and didn't have an increase of unwanted hair, as these are two of the most common visible symptoms of PCOS. In addition to that, I didn't know anyone around me who had it. My mother and sister never had an issue with fertility.

Whether I had an unusual case of PCOS or something else completely different, I was afraid I learned that there are solutions and possible treatments available. There are many women who suffer from it who manage to get pregnant naturally or with a little bit of medical help, but I was still scared

The doctor mentioned ovary stimulation medication that I could take after marriage that should help me get pregnant without further issues. I knew there was something not right in my body. I could feel it, especially since I had ovarian cyst removal surgery when I was seventeen. In my first year of marriage I tried not to think a lot about getting pregnant. I was still only nineteen so we just left it to nature. I wanted to give my body a chance to get pregnant naturally I was so stressed about our new life. Moving to a new country with a new language, culture and climate was enough to deal with

Chapter 2

Marriage and Hope

We enjoyed our first year as a newly married couple. I kept hoping to become pregnant each month as I always wanted to be a mother at young age. I felt that was a great opportunity to grow with your children, to decrease the age gap between mother and child. I wasn't upset when I didn't get pregnant and considered it was due to a bit of delay because of the PCOS. By the second year, I started to visit a new obstetrics and gynecology (OB-GYN) doctor who suggested a couple of tests for both of us. Tests confirmed the PCOS diagnosis, but other than that, we were both healthy and should be able to have children.

My new doctor felt it was just a mild case of PCOS that could be easily improved and would not hinder our attempts to get pregnant. She started me on medication that stimulates the ovaries to produce viable eggs, which I took for six months. The result? Nothing. Not one positive pregnancy test. The only result was bad side effects such as hot flashes and ovarian cysts. We decided to try something else.

After a few months on birth control to regulate my menstrual cycle and to help shrink the ovarian cyst, I started a few cycles of injections to stimulate the ovaries, and I had a better response with this procedure every time. I did have a couple of mature eggs, but for an unknown reason they never made it to pregnancy. I started to panic and fear gripped my heart.

Trying to stay busy, I went back to college to get my associate degree in science, though my bigger dream was to become a mother. But I also wanted to have a better education and future for my children and me. In Palestine, I went to Birzeit University for a year and I took general classes and some specific classes related to law. At that time, I wanted to be lawyer. I don't know why, but I think I was feeling the injustice that comes from living in an occupied country. After I moved to the U.S., I switched my degree to become an elementary educator, as I have a passion for children and education.

We set aside a little more money in savings for future infertility treatments, since we did not have insurance. Treatment is very expensive and was not covered back then. I always wondered why infertility treatments and trying to have a baby is so expensive for some. It seems like many areas in the medical field are expensive, especially for people without insurance. When we did look into health insurance, to my surprise, as soon as I mentioned infertility issues, they refused to cover us. Even the more expensive insurance companies said no. It was frustrating.

Happy third anniversary to us! Time flew (well, not so fast) as we were still waiting for our miracle to happen. I will never forget that long period of waiting and wondering. I can remember a specific doctor's appointment and how I waited patiently for her arrival in the exam room. In a tiny room with all-white décor, I could smell that antiseptic scent of cleaning products. I could hear the telephones ringing, the shuffling of papers, and the sound of footsteps outside the room. This was a scene that I didn't know I would be repeating many, many times in the future—sitting and waiting for a doctor, a procedure, a test, or a test result.

During that visit, my lovely doctor recommended a hysterosalpingogram (HSG) exam to check if there was any blockage to my fallopian tubes. During the process, a dye is injected into the cervix and a thin tube is inserted into the uterus. Then an x-ray is taken which will reveal any abnormalities or blockages in the fallopian tubes. The doctor said it was a very simple process that could be done in an outpatient surgery center.

Even though I kept telling myself it was just an x-ray, the sight of all the nurses and doctors just scared me. My heart felt like it was beating too fast. They gave me a pill that caused me to relax to make the procedure more comfortable. It was very quick and easy, as my doctor said it would be, and the results showed no blockage and normal fallopian tubes. The procedure was not that bad at all. I just felt mild cramping and was feeling great by the end of the day.

I had mixed feelings about the result. I was hoping to find something, at least the reason for the delay. But, on the other hand, it was good to hear that everything was normal. My doctor mentioned that I have a bicornuate uterus, which means my uterus is shaped like a heart. I had never heard of a uterus shaped like a heart. A normal uterus is shaped like an upside-down pear. Mine was not normal, but it should not affect my chances of getting pregnant. The only effect could be early birth, but mine was a very mild case and did not require any further surgeries to fix or correct which was great news and a blessing.

I told myself I would think and worry about all of it later. At that time, I needed to focus on getting pregnant first. If it was not a blockage in the fallopian tubes or the heart shape of the uterus, what else was keeping me from getting pregnant?

We continued the cycle of injections and trigger shots, followed by two weeks of waiting. During those two weeks, I started to feel tired, hungry, and a little different than I had felt after the previous cycles of injections. What was going on with me? Was it what I was thinking? Was I possibly pregnant? I didn't know, but I was scared to get my hopes raised.

I wondered if I should ask Ali to bring home a pregnancy test or if I should just wait for a couple of days. We couldn't take a pregnancy test until two weeks after the trigger shot. Finally, the day came when I could take the test, so I called Ali and asked him to bring the test with him. Sure enough, I was right. I got my very first positive pregnancy test!

That was an amazing feeling. After three long years of tests, shots, and disappointment, I was looking at the two strong lines on the pregnancy test I held in my hand. We had gone through many expensive pregnancy tests in those three years, but this pregnancy test was worth its weight in gold.

Ali was over the moon and he rushed to the phone to tell our families. I knew it was too early to announce the pregnancy, but that's what happened. On the second day, I rushed to my doctor's office and I didn't even call first. I was so excited, but she was not. She scolded me for coming in and taking the test at home, because the result could be related to the hormones in the trigger shot and not an actual pregnancy. Wait, what? It felt like a nightmare possibility and more heartache and disappointment for us.

She recommended that I go home, take another test after two days, and let her know if the lines were getting darker. I was also scheduled for a blood test in four days to confirm the pregnancy. On that day, I felt that my happiness had vanished and I couldn't tell my family that it might be a false positive because they were already so excited. But, as I suspected, it was too early to announce.

I took pregnancy tests daily and the second line was getting darker and clearer each time. With each positive result, my happiness started to kick in again. A blood test confirmed a high level of HCG (human chorionic gonadotropin), which meant we were definitely pregnant.

We were talking about our miracle every day. Ali called multiple times a day from work to check in and ask how I was feeling. I was trying my best to take care of myself. Morning sickness hit me hard, made even worse by the high progesterone supplement I was taking to support the pregnancy. This stress was compounded by the fact that I was in school and it was time for final exams. I was studying intensely to keep my high grades and honor status.

I was able to schedule my classes on two days a week. Having all my classes in two days allowed me more days to study and take care of the household chores. We also had only one car, so Ali would drop me off at college in the morning and I would take public transportation home in the evening.

At seven weeks, we had an appointment to listen to the heartbeat. I could hardly wait! It was such an exciting time. The day before, felt something was off. I was tired bordering on exhausted, and I started to feel strange cramps. I began to feel a wetness and rushed to the bathroom. I was bleeding. I tried to catch my breath and raced to the phone to call Ali. It took a couple of seconds for him to understand the words I tried to say between my crying and shaking voice. I was seven weeks pregnant and bleeding for some unknown reason.

We called my doctor and I was at her clinic within hours. An ultrasound test allowed us to hear that amazing heartbeat still beating strong, but she did see a blood clot near the baby and we prayed that it would pass without harm. Reassured that the baby was still alive, we went home.

At two in the morning, I felt strong pain and cramping that moved from my back to my lower abdominal area. It was enough to wake me up from my sleep. I could barely move my hand to reach Ali. He woke up, startled. His eyes were wide open and he looked terrified. I could barely talk or move. I fainted because my blood pressure was very low and I was bleeding heavily. Ali called the ambulance.

My greatest fear came true as the ultrasound and a blood test confirmed that I lost my baby. I remember repeating that cold, sterile phrase over and over in my head: "lost the baby." Really, they lied to me, because the doctor should have mentioned that I also lost a piece of my soul.

Even though Ali and my family were there to comfort me, I had a deep, hollow space in my heart that only my lost child could fill. In that moment, I felt like the doctors didn't have any empathy and were unprofessional. Was that all they could offer? Cold condolences for our baby? Those words were enough for me to feel as if the world was ending.

Losing a baby at seven weeks was a small, barely noticeable event for the doctors, but to me, it meant the world. The idea of miscarriage never crossed my mind and I didn't want to believe that something like that could happen to me. I thought I already reached my dream to have a child by getting pregnant, but that was not the case. My baby was gone and we were left heartbroken.

It took time for me to get back to normal, mentally and physically. Miscarriage is very hard on a woman's body. If you ask any woman who has dealt with a miscarriage, you will see the tears in their eyes, even though it may have been decades ago. The pain and loss of that child stays with you.

My physical pain was not manageable on my own, and a strong painkiller allowed me to rest and go into a deep sleep. I wanted to sleep so soundly that I wouldn't wake up to reality and be forced to remember that I had lost something that was so precious to me.

The only positive thing that I could think of was that I now knew I could get pregnant. That was a great thing to happen and reassured me, even though the outcome had been so negative. My goal was to get pregnant soon and be able to carry and protect my baby through birth and beyond. Even though the doctors explained that the miscarriage was not my fault, I still felt I didn't protect my child. I felt terrible for days thinking that, as a mother, I couldn't support and protect my baby. Everyone around me tried to raise my hopes up by telling me stories about women who had miscarriages and got pregnant naturally a few cycles afterward. They said it was as if the body just needed to figure out how to get pregnant. Could this happen to me? I hoped so.

Weeks passed and I did not have the same success of those women who became pregnant after a miscarriage. I took a few months' break to give my body time to heal and a chance to get pregnant naturally, as I hoped I could. But that wasn't the reality. It was time to go back to seek further medical options and treatments.

Our hopes were raised when the doctor mentioned the fertility procedure intrauterine insemination (IUI) as a possible route for us. In IUI, the doctor places the sperm inside my uterus to help increase the chance of fertilization. We followed my ovulation cycles very closely and received the treatment on a specific day, followed by the stimulation injections and trigger shot. It was a very straightforward, simple treatment that we were hoping would work. My cousin got pregnant this way with all of her children. I was so excited to try this promising new treatment. I felt like I was close to becoming a mother. I couldn't hide my excitement and Ali shared his excitement, too.

After the IUI procedure, we had another two weeks to wait and see if I was pregnant. Those two weeks were the hardest weeks on me, and my days were filled with nervousness and overthinking. My hopes were high. *This time it will work,* I thought. *I will get pregnant this time.*

I visualized how I should do a pregnancy test alone and make it a surprise, like the pregnancy announcement viral videos I saw on the internet. After two weeks, I did the pregnancy test and waited for the second line to appear. I waited. And waited. It never appeared. I fell down on the bathroom floor crying, and when Ali got home, he knew exactly what the result was when he saw my red eyes, puffy from crying all day. I did three IUI treatments in six months, but each time resulted in a negative outcome that left us both sad and empty.

Chapter 3

Going Home

My OB-GYN seemed to give up, or at least she tried everything that she could do or provide within her education and field. She recommended we try in vitro fertilization (IVF), which meant visiting another fertility clinic that specializes in this type of treatment.

The option seemed promising, but a quick search showed us how expensive it is. We just couldn't afford that kind of treatment. We decided to take a six-month break from everything related to infertility. We celebrated our fifth anniversary together as husband and wife, friends, and as partners together in this journey to try to have a child.

After all of that disappointment, Ali surprised me with two tickets to visit Palestine! It was the first time we would visit Palestine since our move to the U.S. five years before. We missed the days and nights that we used to live here. We missed the family gatherings at our parents' houses and the overall welcoming atmosphere. We were excited to see our friends and family and relax in the familiar setting. But as soon as I set foot in the village, nearly everyone asked me why I didn't have a baby yet.

It was overwhelming and exhausting to keep answering this question. Each new query forced me to explain and re-explain about the fertility treatments and the miscarriage. I was reliving those five years of pain and disappointment with every new question. When I look back, I see I was so immature to think I had to give such complete answers that brought back all the heartache and difficult memories. I should have answered in a polite way that we were trying, and that was it.

IVF treatment became part of the conversation for our extended family. We were surprised to learn the treatment is much cheaper in Palestine than in the U.S. and with a great success rate. For the first time, we started to see it as an option, and this offered us hope. Would this be the answer that gave us our baby? We decided to pursue IVF in Palestine.

The first thing I learned about IVF scared me. I would have to learn to give myself shots every day to stimulate my ovaries to produce the most amount of eggs possible. How could I handle this when I was already scared of needles? Ali always did my injections before with the earlier treatments, but that was only a few shots when compared to the new daily regimen.

We talked about it, decided to move forward with the IVF treatment, and Ali was a big help with the shots. It was miserable having to take these injections, and I often cried for ten minutes afterward. I used an ice pack on my stomach to help numb the area before each injection. Honestly, I didn't know if I was crying because it was hurting me or because I was afraid that the cycle would fail. I had a very deep feeling inside me that this would not work. I think I was preparing myself for failure. I kept telling myself, *Think positive*, but I couldn't resist the very deep feelings of hopelessness. Ali's hopes were up way too high, and he was almost sure of a positive outcome. I didn't know what to think, but we would see whose feelings turned into reality!

The doctors had high expectations also because Ali and I didn't have any real health issues. PCOS is something they don't consider an issue when trying IVF because they will choose the mature eggs and only transfer a good embryo. After ten days of stimulation, my body responded quickly and created mature eggs that were measured in the ultrasound every other day. My stomach was covered in bruises from daily injections. Usually it takes between eight to fourteen days of ovary stimulation to develop healthy eggs.

After the injections, the next step was the egg retrieval. Scared and worried, I sat in the cold operating room waiting for the procedure to start. Egg retrieval, under general anesthesia, is much like it sounds. The process involves inserting a hollow needle and aspirating (suctioning) out the follicles and the eggs. It was a short process and I spent the rest of the day with my new best friends: Cramps, Pain (from the gas inserted to expand my belly like a balloon), and Fatigue.

It was now up to the doctors to combine the viable eggs with my husband's sperm and create each embryo. We waited patiently to hear from them. How many embryos would successfully make it through the process? When would we find out about transferring the eggs into my uterus? Finally, they called and said we had seven embryos that made it to day three. That was a standard milestone for embryos. We would transfer four and freeze three.

On the morning of the embryo transfer, I was ready, though I didn't sleep very well. We drove to the center of Ramallah to the infertility clinic for the transfer. Ramallah is the heart of the West Bank. It is a gorgeous city with very busy roads lined with retail stores and small shops. My favorite area is a big open space with all kinds of organic vegetables for sale. It is like a farmers market in America, only larger and more beautiful. The market brings sellers from many different villages together, and some of the vegetables are grown in the lovely backyard gardens I missed so much. You can you imagine the beautiful sight of all those colors in the rows and rows of fresh vegetables and the wonderful smells of the market and the fresh air.

My favorite spot in the market is where the vendors serve pure, fresh carrot juice that they prepare and pour in front of you to enjoy while walking around before we arrived at the infertility clinic for the transfer. Sipping that juice and walking around the market made me so happy. For five minutes, I was so overjoyed by the possibility of becoming pregnant that I was able to ignore that lingering, deep feeling of failure.

We reached the clinic. We waited a few minutes before they called my name. I said goodbye to Ali and joined three other women in the waiting room who were there for the same procedure. There were four of us, all sharing the same hopes and dreams, in a tiny room with four patient beds. It seemed like infertility took over in this world, as many other couples were also seeking help. Soon, it was my turn to leave the room. I left hearing the other women praying and wishing the best for me.

The moment they transferred the four embryos and showed them to me during the ultrasound was incredible! I was once again holding my babies within me and now it was my responsibility to protect them. Then, another two weeks of waiting until we found it if we were successful. It is the longest two weeks that any woman can go through in the infertility treatment process, and, as I learned earlier, you cannot take a pregnancy test because it will show up positive from the trigger HCG shot. For those two weeks, I stayed at home relaxing and just waiting.

I did have symptoms of pregnancy, and that made me excited, but I knew that the HCG shot could give me the same symptoms. I couldn't keep from getting my hopes up, even though I still had the feeling deep down that the procedure would not work.

Finally, it was the day for blood test to be drawn in order to find out if this cycle was successful or not. Ali was excited; I mean overly excited. I was trying my best to live the moment with him and meet his enthusiasm, but it was hard. In our relationship, he is usually the one with the gut feeling that if often right. I hoped his gut would be right this time, too.

Blood was drawn and we went home to wait for a call. After two hours that felt like a whole day to me and before finishing my dinner, the phone rang and my heart dropped. Ali answered with excitement, but a few seconds later, a pale sadness covered his face. It's enough to say it failed.

Again, after the most extreme procedure I could try, I did not get pregnant. I cried all night when we got the results we were dreading. I asked myself why I was crying because I thought the feeling of failure I had been carrying had prepared me for the negative results. Even though I tried to keep cool and lower my expectations, it still hurt very bad. Nothing can prepare a woman for that kind of heartache and disappointment, even if you try not to get your hopes up and think you can handle it.

No explanation whatsoever. It just didn't happen. Overall, the success rate is only 25 percent each time. The doctor said we could try again with the three frozen embryos. She said many women do great with this and have a successful pregnancy. Despite my sadness, I still felt excited and agreed with the doctor. I whispered to Ali, "Let me try this." At least there were fewer needles this time and one more cycle couldn't hurt. We didn't have to go through the ovary stimulation process or the egg retrieval. We waited for another month and we were ready for embryo transfer We did the transfer of the three remaining embryos and waited another two weeks. What did we have to lose?

During that waiting period, my husband had to fly back to the U.S. He had to go back to work and couldn't stay any longer. We also had already spent a lot of money. I stayed with family in our lovely village, waiting and waiting. It was harder than last time since Ali had left. I missed him so much. *What if this cycle fails again and I have to face it by myself?* I wondered.

Finally, the day arrived for the blood test to detect pregnancy. I would now learn if this cycle was a success or just another failure. I did not have any symptoms, which I had since learned not to focus on because in this stage they don't mean anything.

The nurse took the blood sample and asked me to come back within an hour. I left the clinic and took a walk in the middle of Ramallah, drank my favorite fresh carrot juice, and walked back to the clinic after that hour, an hour that felt like four hours. Usually time flies so fast, but with the waiting, it just got slower. I took a seat in the waiting room praying to my Allah inside of my heart and trying to calm down by taking deep breaths.

"Neveen." They called me to come up to the check-in window. The young lady was holding an envelope between her hands. My heart dropped to the floor, but her smile gave me peace. She whispered,

"Congratulations! You are pregnant! HCG blood came in at 95. We recommend repeating it after a week, but we consider anything above 25 to indeed be pregnant."

Oh, I was so excited, but nervous too. I wished Ali was there, but it was too late to call him. It was 3:00 a.m. in Chicago which meant he was probably sleeping, but I wanted to call. I needed to call. I couldn't handle the excitement, so I rang his number and woke him up with the news. He answered the phone and I screamed "I'm pregnant!" I think I heard him crying. He was over the moon once again.

One week passed and I repeated the test. This time it came back with an HCG level at 1700. Oh, my God! That was a great increase and a positive sign. The same day, I started bleeding and called the doctor. The doctor said it should be OK and that happened sometimes, especially with IVF. They recommended I stay on my medication and repeat the blood test in a few days.

My hormone level raised a little, and it seemed promising, but I still had a sense that something was not right. There was more spotting and that made me terrified to go visit my doctor for another test. The new blood test showed a decrease in HCG levels. I couldn't believe it. What was going on?

Then they told me, "Sorry, it seemed to be a chemical pregnancy."

"Excuse me, what does that even mean? Are you playing with my emotions?" I asked.

"Ma'am, we are sorry, but there is no baby," the doctor said solemnly.

This was devastating. After seven embryos and two cycles of IVF, each failed attempt was harder and harder to get over. After a few days, I was done crying. I decided to fly back to Chicago. This cycle killed me. It broke my spirit.

Chapter 4

Back to Square One

Four weeks later, I was sitting on my comfortable sofa looking through the window outside. It was spring in Chicago and I love spring. It is a new soul added to mine. Spring is for hope. It is knowing that the trees and plant you see outside will rebloom, even if you thought the beauty of nature would never live again or survive after the harsh winter. I lit my favorite lavender candle and sat in my comfortable pajamas. I worried, I wondered, and I asked myself, *What else can I try to get pregnant?*

Searching through my laptop, I came across a website advertising herbs that claimed one particular herb was great for infertility. *Should I try it?* I thought. Why not? What did I have to lose?

I ordered some through the website and, once it arrived in the mail, I gave it a try. For two months, I had very bad headaches and cramping. The side effects were so severe that I had to stop. Herbs are like medications. You cannot just take it without consulting a specialist, I learned.

During this time, I also researched acupuncture. It is supposed to help, and despite my fear of needles, I gave it a try. A couple of months later, no results. Perhaps it was time to reconsider infertility treatments.

The IVF process in America seemed promising. A clinic we looked into had better equipment and more extensive testing if we needed it. It was expensive and took us two years to save the $25,000 that was required. That was steep compared to $5,000 in Palestine. We visited the clinic for the first time and found it to be very big, fancy, and clean. They reviewed my file that I sent through email and asked for a test that cost thousands of dollars in our first visit. They ordered medication for another $10,000 and we were ready to start.

This time, the doctor requested a CA-125 blood test that checked to see if I had endometriosis. This was a new phrase to me. "Endo" is a disorder where tissue that should grow inside of the uterus also grows outside of the uterus in areas such as ovaries and fallopian tubes. Severe endometriosis can be painful. My test came back positive and indicated a mild case of endometriosis, even though I learned later on that the blood tests are not always accurate when checking for endometriosis. We had a meeting with the doctor to discuss the results.

Even though it seemed I did have mild endo, he recommended we keep going through the process of IVF because the two should not affect each other. I took a deep, frustrated breath and wondered, *Then why did you request this $300 test if it didn't make a difference?* I gave him the benefit of the doubt and figured he may have needed that information for medication or something like that. I was glad I waited for him to finish before I said anything because he then told me that due to the endo I would be on a high dose of blood thinner to help with implantation of the embryos.

The process was essentially the same as before. The only difference was I got my private room. Again, another two weeks to wait.

After egg retrieval and embryo transfer, I started to experience bloating that made me look five months pregnant. I could barely move from the pain. I went to the doctor again and was diagnosed with Ovarian Hyperstimulation Syndrome (OHSS). OHSS is a condition where the ovaries become extremely swollen from the ovary stimulation IVF medication. It can build up fluid around the abdomen, which was what happened to me. The only good thing about it was that worsening OHSS is sometimes a sign that the embryo attached and pregnancy occurred. I had to monitor myself closely and check my weight daily to see if I needed to go to emergency room to drain the fluid. I was desperately hoping the OHSS would be worth it and we would be successful this time. I started to raise my hopes high. Very high.

A short time later, I felt much better and I knew a pregnancy test was only a few days away. I was so excited! How could I not let the excitement get to my heart, especially knowing that many women who experience OHSS end up being pregnant? We had transferred two embryos and the day came to have a blood test and home pregnancy test. *What if they both implanted?* I wondered. *I would love to have twins.* Actually, it was one of my dreams to be a mother of twins. I knew twins would be twice the work, but I would take it.

Ali was so excited he could hardly wait until the test, too. He brought home a pregnancy test to take in the early morning before heading to the clinic to do the blood test. The result was negative. My heart dropped and I felt like I was this was not happening. On the way to the clinic, I kept hoping that the home pregnancy test was expired or defective in some way. I searched online and read about how other women had negative home pregnancy test results because their HCG levels were not high enough for a home pregnancy test to pick when they were, in fact, pregnant. Could I be one of them?

I waited patiently for the phone call from the clinic that was supposed to come around 4:00 p.m. The phone rang and I felt numb when they said, "I am sorry. Your result is negative." After that call, I felt the weight of the world heavy on my chest. Crying was the only thing that I could do at that moment and through the hours that followed.

The doctor was sorry that we didn't get the result we hoped for and, as before, had no explanation whatsoever about this failure. However, he still thought that IVF was the only option for us since my PCOS was getting worse and worse. Even with PCOS, they still considered us in the category of "unexplained infertility" because of the IVF failure and our relatively good health overall. Having a good grade embryo to transfer is the main factor for successful implantation.

I felt sorry for Ali. Not just because we got a negative result, but also because of the amount of money we were spending on treatment. The treatment in America cost five times more than the amount of money we paid in Palestine. By this time, we had three failed attempts at IVF. After the emotional disappointment and the financial punch we took, we needed a long break to recover from our losses. No more IVF in the U.S. for us. It was too expensive. We decided to go back to Palestine for a while.

Another visit to our beautiful country was upon us. Ali and I started to build a house there. We had been saving for years and were so excited to have our first home together, one we could build the way we wanted. We put ourselves on a limited monthly budget to save for this, and we skipped the IVF treatments for two years to reach another long-term goal and build the house.

It is a large house with three stories. The first floor has a huge kitchen with a big island in the middle like the ones you may see on TV shows. The family room has a fireplace where we can burn wood on cold days. The living room, dining room, and spacious guest bathroom are great spaces for gathering with family and friends. It seems like a big house for two people, and I can hear other people saying that while walking around the house. It hurts not to have children to fill our beautiful home.

We chose beige flooring with dark brown cabinets that give the feeling of a comfy, classic, chic look. The second story is my favorite. It is a combination of our master suite with the king bed, spacious bath, walk-in closet, office, and a balcony. We turned another family room into a library to study and read, and there's also a spacious terrace, two big bedrooms, and a bathroom in between for our children. The last story has a guest bedroom with a bath and a huge terrace that has a priceless view of the mountains, plains, the green trees, and the neighboring homes in the village. I often go up there just to breathe the fresh air and relax.

I always wanted a big family. I have six siblings and Ali has nine. Both families are close and it is amazing how we have a great relationship where we love and support each other. I always hoped for my children to be the same. I want them to grow up with that closeness and know their grandparents, aunts, uncles, and cousins.

As soon as we stepped into our home, we started talking about going to Ramallah to visit the IVF clinic and create a plan because we were only staying for short time this visit. I started the IVF process (this was round four) and nine years of trying. This time I wasn't scared of needles or the operating room like before. I was starting to get used to it. I even gave myself the shots as I felt more in control. Then we waited another two weeks, paying attention to my body and hoping that it might give me a clue to what was going on. Three days before I could test, I started to bleed heavily. My heart was back in that discouraged place and I thought it was another failure. I was right.

Since we already had a frozen embryo, we decided to transfer it during the next cycle. Just like before, Ali had to leave me to fly back to America. I stayed there, facing this failure by myself. Did I say failure? Yes. Round five was officially added to the list of unsuccessful IVF attempts. This time, I was angry, crushed, and demanded an explanation. My poor doctor asked me to calm down while she ran to get the big boss.

The doctor who established the clinic has a wealth of knowledge and experience. I asked him for an explanation and a solution, but he didn't have one. Or at least I wished he hadn't said the option that he did. He told me that it might just be that Ali and I could not have children together. He was saying that although we were both healthy, and nothing in particular was wrong, for some reason, we couldn't conceive a child.

This blew my mind. *How dare you mention this! No thank you. I will pass on your advice.* I didn't completely get over this idea of giving up. It stayed in my brain for a while and was killing me every time I thought about it. *Why, Ali and I have the best relationship any couple could hope for. This doctor! He must be out of his mind.*

Chapter 5

Our Next Move?

As the most recent loss continued to ache, I found myself sitting on our home terrace, wiping my tears, when a strange idea came to my mind. What about Jordan? As Palestinians, we aren't allowed to travel through the one airport in our area, so when traveling, we must first cross the border into Jordan and fly out of the Jordanian airport. There is a fertility clinic in Jordan and I knew a couple of women who had successful IVF from there. The idea alone brought joy to my tired soul. I wasn't ready to give up. Why not have a consultation since I was going to be in Jordan soon anyway?

After four weeks I reached my destination in Jordan and visited the clinic. The first impression was great and the staff were very professional. First, I met with one doctor who did the basic exam and ultrasounds. I was clear that if they could provide me with any additional treatment, I will go further and start the process. I wasn't going to do the basic IVF that I already did several times.

After a very long day, with five doctors looking over my case, they suggested a new IVF cycle with intracytoplasmic sperm injection, known as ICSI. Basically, it meant they would inject a healthy sperm into a mature egg for a better chance of fertilization. All of my previous IVF attempts were done without this technology. We decided to move forward. It seemed promising, and within twenty days, we did the egg retrieval. This would mark round six of IVF and our third procedure in three months.

Ali arrived in Jordan to join me in this process. It wasn't hard to convince him to try again, as he was just as desperate for a child as I was. Having him there made my life shine. Thankfully, my aunt and her family lived in Jordan and we had a great time with them. On the day of the embryo transfer, I realized this was the first time I was excited about embryo transfer in many years. I had hope. Everything seemed to move smoothly as planned. Even though we only retrieved seven eggs, five of them made it to three days, which was a good milestone for embryos. All five embryos had great A and B grades, which meant that our chances for a successful implantation were good.

This time they tried new medication to help with implantation. The doctors decided to transfer five embryos. That's is a lot in one cycle, but we were hoping one or two would make it. They even used a special glue to attach the embryos to my uterus. This was new for me. I was so excited. This was going to be the one, I could just feel it.

The only concern the doctors raised was what if all the embryos attached? They told me if that happened, I would need to do a process where they remove one or two embryos to give the others a better chance to survive. *There's no way I can do that*, I thought, but I shook my head and said, "Let's see how many will implant first." I didn't want to consider that possibility.

My doctors said that it would be fine to travel back to the U.S. over that two-week period. Two weeks after the transfer, it was safe to do a pregnancy test which I assumed it was positive. I wanted to surprise Ali, even though he told me not to do the test without him. But it seemed I hadn't learned my lesson because I was desperate to surprise him and record his reaction on video. My mind told me, *This one is the one! I am positive! I can feel it. I am pregnant!* The day of the test, he was making his coffee to leave for work and he asked me to wait until he got back so we could do it together.

I couldn't wait and rushed into the bathroom to take the test before he even left for work. I wanted to surprise him like I had always imagined. I did the pregnancy test and waited for the second line. And waited. The test was negative. Not even a faint line. This cycle was another failure. He came running upstairs when he heard my loud, painful cries. How did I feel so certain and knew I could feel it? It seems sometimes our feelings are what we are hoping for, and we want them to be real.

Three in vitro cycles in a row left my body noticeably weak and tired. When I think about it right now, I feel sad and angry at myself. I was so desperate to have a baby that I didn't think about what I did to my body. Putting my body through those consequent cycles was the craziest thing I ever did and I needed time to heal physically and mentally. I decided to give myself a good long break and planned a quick trip to Palestine for twenty days. But this time, I was not seeking infertility treatment. No more needles. No more disappointment. I just wanted to enjoy being around the family.

I wanted to visit Jerusalem, as it had been a long time since I had been there. During that time, someone mentioned a very good doctor who may be able to help us. Despite my plans to relax and not think about having a baby, I called the doctor's office. No one answered, but I figured I would just walk in, as most of our clinics are walk-ins. This time for consultation only. I was not ready for another IVF attempt.

Jerusalem always moves me on a very deep level. Looking at the golden color of the Dome of the Rock, I can feel the hidden emotions inside me. The place is very sacred and holy for us as Muslims. Making my prayers and *duaa* inside the mosque truly brings peace and hope into my heart. In Jerusalem, people from the mosques and churches hug each other. After the *athan* (the Islamic call to prayer) is sounded from the mosque, the church bells will play.

The streets of Jerusalem tell their own story as believers and tourists from all over the world have visited for centuries. I am sure no one was looking at Jerusalem as I did that day. After my visit and prayers in the

Dome of the Rock, I went to search for that doctor. I asked a couple of people for directions, and once I reached my destination, I discovered the office was closed. I wasn't too sad about it. At least I had an amazing visit and, honestly, I didn't think this clinic would have anything new to add to my case. I went back to my small village and tried my best to just enjoy my visit. On the last day, we said goodbye to our families and friends and flew back to America.

Months passed and we lived our lives full of love and with our eyes focused on success. We were still trying to have a baby and did pregnancy tests every month. The key was that we were still happy together as a couple. My friend mentioned a great doctor that her sister went to who helped her become pregnant after years of trying. Why not? I called and scheduled an appointment. I went to that office by myself and met the new doctor. After a quick ultrasound, she shook her head.

"Your ovaries are like an old lady! PCOS is severe, natural pregnancy almost impossible, and you have a very minimal chance of success," she said with a strange boldness.

I opened my eyes wide and took a deep breath. She was honest, straight forward, and it shocked me. "I can't help you with anything," she said. And when I mentioned to her how many IVF rounds I went through, she took a minute of silence and then asked why I was doing this to my body.

"Just give up having a baby or seek IVF with a donor egg," she said.

"I can't," I replied. "I am a Muslim and this is not allowed it as it is basically another woman's DNA. At least from my point of view, I want a child who carries my DNA and looks like me and my husband."

I left the office empty-handed and felt that the whole world was pressing down hard on me. Once I reached my house and laid on my couch, I didn't cry. Even though I wanted to, there were no tears to drop. *I will keep trying. There must be a solution. Allah will lead me to it.*

To change my mood, I went to the kitchen and cooked our favorite meal. I was trying to switch my negative thinking and put my energy into something that brings a smile to us. I cooked a Middle Eastern meal called *maqluba*. If I wanted to translate that name in English, it is basically upside down. It is a dish of cooked meat, rice, and fried vegetables placed in one pot. When it is time for serving, we flip the pot upside down on to a large plate and that's where the unique name comes from.

As soon as Ali entered the house, he knew what was for dinner as the delicious smell was stronger than the scent of my lavender candle. We both sat to enjoy our meal and suddenly, he asked how my appointment was. I shared the experience with Ali and told him what the doctor said in detail.

This was the first time he didn't say anything. Not a word. *Is he giving up on having children with me?* I wondered, and the thoughts kept coming. *Has his patience run out? I don't blame him, but this is not my choice either. Am I overthinking right now? Will he leave me to remarry in order to have children? What am I going to do?* I was just so depressed, discouraged, and I felt lost and broken.

Chapter 6

Another Chance

I started working as an elementary teacher's assistant. The first-grade students gave me positive energy every day with their loving and caring attitudes. They were so sweet to be around, even though it was sometimes challenging to manage twenty young children at the same time.

While chatting with one of my co-workers during our lunch break, I mentioned my struggle with infertility. She told me that our district insurance covered IVF treatments. Really? I felt excitement in my heart. I had never asked about that and never even thought it would be a possibility. It turned out that my insurance not only covered one, but four, attempts. That was great news, however, insurance did not cover the medication for the treatment, which was around $13,000. I talked to my Ali about it, and together we came up with a plan to go further.

That meant I could try another IVF treatment and it would be covered by insurance! I thought I had given up on doing any more fertility treatments. *No, I am not done. I will keep seeking my dream.* We searched for the best clinic in Illinois and ended up in a great clinic with the most amazing, down-to-earth, professional staff. The doctor listened intently to our concerns and questions. He suggested that since this would be our seventh attempt, I should also do genetic testing.

On the day of the testing, thirteen blood samples were taken and I began to get dizzy. I woke up after I fainted, with one of the nurses holding an icepack on my neck and forehead. After the results came in, the doctor decided he wanted us to try the long protocol. This meant I would take birth control for a month and then start with a menstrual cycle and injections to stimulate the ovaries.

I took the list of medications needed and called the pharmacy. They came back with estimates of $14,000, which was even more than we had planned on. In addition, while my tests were covered by insurance, any tests related to Ali would have to be paid out of pocket. This was over our budget and we could not afford it. I didn't know what to do next. Should I call the clinic and cancel my follow-up appointment and try to save money for a couple of months? This seemed promising and I wanted to try it as soon as possible. We needed to make this a priority.

I called Ali and asked him if he knew of any pharmacists who might have the medication for less money. He told me he would ask a friend of his who worked in the medical field. Ali called me back and told me that his friend knew a pharmacist who may be able to help, but they needed the medication list to send us an estimate. If we could save a couple thousand dollars, we could at least cover Ali's tests, too.

I was cooking in my small kitchen with light Arabic music playing in the background. The smell of roasted chicken filled the room as I prepared dinner when suddenly the phone rang.

"Hello, my love! Guess what?" asked Ali.

"What is it? Tell me," I responded.

"Can you figure the cost estimate the new pharmacy gave us? Take a guess."

"I can't guess, but your voice seems happy and excited. What is the cost?" I asked.

"FREE!"

"Free? What do you mean free?" I asked. I couldn't figure out what he was saying. How were these expensive medications suddenly free?

He told me that the pharmacy owner and his wife were trying to get pregnant for a while. They decided to do in vitro, and they even prepared everything and purchased the medication to start. But, for some reason, they didn't begin the treatment and she got pregnant naturally that month. They were about to take the medications to their clinic to donate when we called at the exact right time.

I couldn't believe him. In the beginning, I thought he was just saying this to make it easier on me. *Maybe he was borrowing most of the money from his friend*, I whispered to myself. But he told me he would get the pharmacy number so I could call the wife and thank her.

When I made the call, she told me the same story my husband had given me. We received most of the medication we needed, and I sent her flowers to thank her for her generosity. Their kind act meant we could move forward with the process.

I took all my medications and my body responded positively. I had fifteen mature eggs that were ready for egg retrieval. I felt swollen and my stomach looked like I was five months pregnant. It was a great relief after the process was over, and now we took a break for a month while my embryos reached seven days maturity before freezing.

While my body had time to recover, my mind was still thinking about it every long day. Only two embryos made it to day seven. I was expecting more, but it was OK. Those two were probably the strongest ones. The doctor gave us the choice to transfer one or two. We decided to go with two to increase our chances, and if they both implanted, that would be great.

Back at work, it was nearly spring break at the school. The students were always very excited before breaks. By "excited" I mean playing around when they were supposed to be reading and chatting with others about their plans when they were supposed to be listening to the teacher. They were running around all over the place. I was used to being on my feet all day, but on that day, I felt exhausted like I was hit by a train. I was very tired and just wanted to get home and lie down. I was so tired that I almost forgot that today was also the day I could take the pregnancy test, which I did.

Positive! Two clear strong lines!

We were beyond excited! We were pregnant again with a blood test to confirm it. I needed an ultrasound at six weeks to hear the baby's heartbeat. We were thrilled and wondered if one baby attached or if they both did. I would love to have twins.

We walked to the clinic for our ultrasound, excited to find out more. The ultrasound technician took a while looking and measuring, but she didn't say anything. I asked what she could see, and she said she could only see the sac but nothing in it. They asked me to come back the following week. Hopefully, they could see the baby then, because sometimes it is a little too early. Imagine what that week was like! It was a very painful, stressful, and anxious week that seemed to last forever. When enough time had passed, I walked to the clinic again feeling less fear and anxiety this time, but not the same excitement of the previous appointment.

When the ultrasound was over, there was no baby.

In addition to the sad news, I was diagnosed with a blighted ovum. Blighted ovum is when the embryo attaches to the uterine wall but does not develop further, even though the hormone HCG is processed by cells in the placenta and displays a positive pregnancy test. My doctor recommended stopping all medication in order to let my body get it out it naturally. Unfortunately, I had to do a dilation and curettage (D&C) procedure where tissue and the remnants of the pregnancy are scooped from the uterus.

This was my third time doing a D&C after each miscarriage. There is something unique about my body that does not get rid of the remnants of the pregnancy naturally. It is as if my body wants the baby so much and tries so hard to keep it. I felt like I was close to giving up, but I held myself together. Reading inspirational stories about other women who dealt with infertility was my way to keep my motivation up.

It was my 31st birthday and I had lost my baby three weeks before. I was still trying to get it over it physically and emotionally. I know it's true that 31 is a relatively young age, and I still had time to have a baby, but the fact that I had been trying for years was scary.

Ali came home that day holding a small bag with my birthday gift inside. He got me an airplane ticket for a two-week vacation with my parents and brother that would return me to the Middle East and visit few countries in the way. I was so happy! It had been a long time since I had spent time with my parents. Of course, I wished he could join us, but he couldn't due to his work schedule. At least, that was what I thought.

I started to believe he wanted to try taking break from each other. I thought he mostly wanted some time to see if he could go further in life without me. No matter the reason, I was so grateful and thankful for his gift. Also, it can be beneficial to occasionally have some time apart in married life. The trip was an opportunity for us to realize the value of our marriage and life together. And it was hard to even spend two weeks apart. His daily calls, messages, and overall attitude showed me that we can't live far away from each other, even though we were still seeking a big dream that seemed hard to reach as a couple.

Taking vacations and visiting new places was also a great remedy to heal my body and mind, since our financial situation had improved and we could seek more treatments. A quick trip with my parents and brother was like a balm for my soul. And it began in France.

Chapter 7

A Shift in Thinking

Standing in Paris on a windy March day, a cup of hearty espresso in my hand while I gazed at the Eiffel tower, was a great mind detox. After our stop in France, we headed to Palestine, spent a few days there, and continued our trip to Egypt. Pyramids and the unique artifacts amazed me. I had seen them before in pictures, but seeing ancient Egypt in real life was breathtaking. After a long day visiting the best and must-see places in Cairo, we headed to Turkey.

Istanbul is beautiful, and it contains a hidden magnetism that pulls you to stay there. It's a city with a perfect mix of cultures between the European and Middle Eastern traditions at their best. Taking a walk through the Galata Bridge and seeing the old and new buildings made happiness swell inside my heart. Two weeks of traveling had a profound positive impact on my tired mind. I came back with a fresh outlook and renewed hope.

Back in Chicago, I rejoined with Ali at our "home sweet home." I finished the school semester and said goodbye to my lovely students. It was time to enjoy summer after a year full of work, IVF treatments, miscarriages, and, of course, some amazing days full of blessings. This year we were going to spend the beautiful summer back home to Palestine.

Time passed and we celebrated our thirteenth wedding anniversary in Palestine surrounded by family and friends we loved dearly. We were blessed to be in our own Palestinian home and, as with every previous visit, this one brought something new. We heard from an old friend that there was a fertility clinic nearby that was using a new IVF protocol, and its high rate of success seemed very promising. We decided to try again. What else could we do?

The first fresh cycle produced great grade-level embryos for implantation and the doctors seemed excited. The familiar two-week waiting time passed but resulted in yet another negative pregnancy test. I still had three frozen embryos the doctor recommended we transfer, so we did. I waited another two stressful weeks. This was two transfers in two months. Again, the test was negative. I usually consider myself to be a strong woman. I was brave enough to move to America. I've struggled through infertility and handled years' worth of disappointment. This time, I was truly done. I was tired, exhausted, and heartbroken.

This round broke me. Totally. I gave up and needed a couple of days of crying alone to get all my anger and sadness out. My body was done with all the injection bruises and tenderness. I was finished. I asked people to please not mention in vitro or fertility treatments ever again. But I knew that if I don't get what I want, I need to seek another way to reach my goal. It was time for transformation. In the Quran, Allah says, "the Almighty changes the fate of no people unless they themselves show a will for change." I needed to change, and I would find the way to reach my dream.

I love traveling and exploring a new culture, language, and cuisine. We had visited a couple of countries so far, but my wish or must-visit list was growing every day. I enjoy traveling, walking through the airports, and shopping from the duty-free, which many women will agree on.

However, every time we visited a country, the idea of infertility and visiting specialty clinics controlled our stay. I was sitting in the Amman airport heartbroken, having my American coffee and thinking, *What have I done all these years and what is left to do? Is there something I haven't tried yet?* Fourteen years is a long time to walk the same path and still not reach your destination. The idea of changing my lifestyle came across my mind. This thought began to take shape within me. As I sat there, I could think of nothing else. The idea of change controlled me. For the first time, I didn't even check the duty-free stores or walk around. I was busy thinking.

I believe in Allah and I pray to him daily to show me the way. It seemed that I had to find another path to reach my goal. But how could I find that way? Where would I start, who would I follow, and what did I need to change? I decided to invest in myself, to educate myself, and improve my ways of dealing with infertility.

I was tired of having heartbroken episodes, being sensitive to baby-related subjects, and crying for days. I turned my focus to me, to my body and my mind. I never believed in self-development courses and exercises, but this time I would give it a try. I could both improve myself and learn how to deal with infertility and reach my goal to become a mother. I started to search online, typing keywords like "infertility solutions," "success stories with medical alternatives," and "how to be a better person."

Chapter 8

Taking Responsibility

"You are responsible for what happens to you." Dr. Ahmed Emara, spoken in an internet video about responsibility.

These words fell on my ears like a sonic boom. How could I be responsible for not having children even though we had been trying for fourteen years and had exhausted all the fertility options we could think of? I did every process known to medicine and still didn't have a baby. Was that my responsibility? I still hadn't reached my dream. I can take responsibility for my life, decisions, work, and relationships, but how could I be responsible for not having children?

I watched a video online from Dr. Ahmed Emara who specialized in human health and development. That was all that I needed to wake up from the longest nightmare that anyone trying to get pregnant could have. Dealing with infertility, any chronic medical condition, or just seeking to reach your dream (that takes forever) is painful and hard, and sometimes you just take the easiest road and give up. Now Dr. Emara was telling me that I am also responsible for not reaching my dream to become a mother. It was a revelation.

Once I got over that confusing feeling of blame and responsibility, I couldn't resist watching more online videos and courses. In a couple of days I watched ten of the videos on the internet. I listened to them while cooking, cleaning, and driving. Every video led to another one, each with a focus on motivation and life development skills. I felt like this was what my soul was looking for. His words about motivation and creating a stress-free life were very hopeful for my tired body and mind. Within days, I invested an additional half an hour from my day to watch, learn, and take notes about these new self-development skills.

In the beginning, I was skeptical about it. I thought that self-development skill lectures and exercises sounded ideal but were far away from reality and hard to apply. *But, hey! I have nothing to lose. I will give this a try*, I whispered to myself.

I started taking responsibility for my life and I stopped complaining about anything that was going on around me. I stopped complaining about my irregular cycle, polycystic ovary syndrome, and endometriosis. I was responsible for anything that might pop up in my life: not my husband, not my family, not my boss, not the community. Just ME.

I needed to learn that no words or actions hurt me without my permission. I would protect my heart, emotions, and overall life. No one would come and save, help, or guide me. Taking charge helped me raise my self-esteem because my life was now in my hands. I could shape it the way I wanted and live it the way I wanted. I took responsibility for my physical and mental health. As a result, I started to feel stronger and more confident.

After I took responsibility and applied these principles to my life, it was time to do my homework and research. No one was going to just magically appear and help me reach my goal. Reading books was my first option. For an average cost of $15 per book, I had an instant mentor that could educate me and share their years of experience. I don't have enough years to try everything by myself, so learning through the stories of others added to my knowledge and experience. I learned mistakes to avoid and read about other peoples' challenges, failures, and successes.

The second option was taking an online course. Sometimes these courses can be expensive, but for me, they were worth every penny. I specifically searched for the teachings of anyone who had reached the goal I wanted to reach. Which, in my case, was any woman who finally became a mother after years of unexplained infertility. The internet is a great invention! You can find out any kind of information there.

My research brought me to a woman who lives in Sydney and her story inspired me and gave me hope. I learned about Dr. Gabriela Rose and her natural fertility breakthrough program where she first helped herself and, eventually, helped women all over the world overcome their infertility. Her books and courses were my first stop. Then it was all on my end to practice and do even more research and, most importantly, to find the best way to support what my body needed to get pregnant. I spent a lot of time searching "unexplained infertility" because I believed that there was something in my body that was refusing to carry a baby, a conclusion I came to after all our failed in vitro attempts.

I put myself in charge of understanding my body. Our bodies are amazing creations that give us signs and symptoms that sometimes only we can figure out. I started to listen to my body and take better care of it. I researched more about what I ate and found ways to manage my stress level. Irregular menstrual cycles and spotting between cycles mean something is off. My body was trying to tell me something and I needed to figure out what it was.

All my reading about diets and best practices in nutrition led me to stop eating sugar. I put together a new Lifestyle Notebook where I took notes on all my findings and important facts. After I wrote down the recommendation to stop eating sugar, I started to write down my food intake that included any sugar. My morning coffee contained one teaspoon of sugar. My snacks contained sugar. My evening dessert was sugary. The list just kept on growing. I discovered that sugar was a prominent element in my diet that I needed to replace and remove completely.

I stopped eating sugar and limited my foods to natural-based sugar sources. The first two weeks were hard and miserable. I craved sugar all the time. If my craving was strong, I would take one piece of fruit or dried fruit, like my favorite, dried figs. I fought myself every time I walked to the pantry for a piece of chocolate and instead made a better choice, such as raw almonds.

After three weeks, the cravings stopped and my body was feeling awesome. I felt lighter, had more energy, had glowing skin, and my next menstrual cycle had less pain. I took this as a good sign that meant my body was trying to tell me to stop eating sugar. My new diet affected Ali, too. We started to snack healthier and switched our nightly dessert to better choices, such as homemade popcorn with coconut oil.

It was time to add to this healthier lifestyle after I found that there is a link between gluten products and infertility. Even if this information was not 100 percent accurate or there is incomplete research on the connection, I decided to do my own experiment. I wasn't losing anything by eliminating gluten products from my diet. Some people do that to detox and clean the system after years of gluten that our body stores. It wasn't hard to stop eating gluten since there is gluten-free bread widely available in stores that I could use for my sandwiches. I loved my new lifestyle and I started to notice that I ate even more vegetables than before, which was great.

My typical day started with at least three cups of coffee with caffeine. *Is it too much? I think it may not be healthy for infertility. Should I give this a try and limit it? This is a hard one for me. How I can start my day without my cup of coffee?* I wondered. *Well, let's make everything right and let's take this time to clean my body.* Not drinking coffee was tough, but not impossible. I made it despite the headache for the first few days. I started to decrease my intake and finally managed to stop completely. Starting my day with warm water and a lemon was great for my body. Two weeks later, I forget all about coffee and loved my caffeine-free teas.

Dairy is another hot topic that healthy lifestyle websites often talk about. They say it is full of hormones that are not really great for your body. I never liked dairy. I don't eat cheese daily, so I was fine to cut it out completely, including yogurt. It had been a while since I drank milk and I switched to almond milk because I feel bloated after I eat dairy, especially ice cream, or drink cow's milk. Was bloating a sign of an allergy? I had never considered it.

My main goal for these changes was to stick to this strict diet and healthier lifestyle and try to clean my body after years of unhealthy food choices. I also started to try alternative natural pregnancy booster remedies. I would say that I put myself under my own experimental research. Why not? Nothing I was doing was dangerous or had side effects. I was eating natural foods and detoxing my body.

I also learned about the importance of infertility massage, which is a great way to increase blood to my ovaries. I did it by myself. After my menstrual cycle ended, I would lie down and do a circle massage on my uterus. Ten times to the right in a circular motion and then ten times to the left. I did that for five days, three times a day, on an empty stomach. Basically, before I got up in the morning, before lunch, and at bedtime. I could feel a difference and knew this massage was helping with the blood flow. During this time, I was trying my best to stay away from medical treatment. I wasn't against medical treatments or IVF. I did nine rounds and many other couples have had successful results through IVF. I knew it worked, but I couldn't make that my focus at that time.

I planned to take six months to a year and prepare my body to get pregnant naturally. If I didn't, I would seek medical treatment to help boost my chances. Until then, I wanted to prepare my body and maximize the possibility of a pregnancy. Round nine, the last attempt at in vitro, had been the hardest. I was not done with my dream, but I was done with IVF for now.

If the IVF had been our best option, we would have had a baby by that point. I think I was immature to keep trying the same process and expecting new results. Dr. Emara once said that you can achieve any goal you want, and the only two things that hold you back are wrong information or missing information. I needed more information.

Chapter 9

Self-Reflection

I want to take a moment out of my story to emphasize how big of a change I encountered when I started taking responsibility for my life. I wish I had known this secret of success years ago. This would have helped me weather the painful moments that I went through every time I failed with IVF.

Taking responsibility was the first skill to learn and apply to my life. Imagine you were in a ship and there was more than one captain and they were arguing about the ship's destination. One captain thinks the ship should head north and the other wants to go south. Would you be fine with that? Do you think they will each reach their desired destination? If they keep doing this, it will take a longer time to reach the destination, if they ever reached it at all.

Don't give your ship (life) to anyone else. You are the captain. Taking responsibility is a life-changing event and a true turning point. Your life is in your hands and you are the one who is responsible for it. Do yourself a favor and stop complaining about others. It is your problem in the first place if you are not having a happy life. That is because of you, and if you are having any other underlying issues in your life, it is also because of you. You are the only one who can change your life.

Avoid lying. We need to be completely be honest with ourselves and others, no matter the consequences. So many problems come from the lies we tell ourselves and others to avoid anxiety and punishment. This always ends up making the situation worse and turns it into a bigger issue. Be brave and take responsibility for your mistakes. That is how we improve and learn. If you lie, you will fool your brain and convince yourself that false truths are reality. Your life will only grow more complicated.

Taking charge of my life is the first step that I took to achieve my dream of becoming a mom. It could be a silly dream for others, but for me, it was the whole world. Having children can be effortless and natural for some, but not for everyone. There are many people around us suffering silently from infertility. In my case, I spent fourteen years trying to get pregnant and endured nine failed IVF treatments. I traveled to a couple of countries to try new techniques and spent thousands of dollars on medication and tests. No matter what your dream is, taking charge of your life is the first step to take to seek your goal.

I was about to give up on my dream, especially because everyone around us started urging us to accept the reality and save our money and effort. However, because this is MY life, I will keep seeking and never let go of my dreams. I will never give up.

We did consider other options such as adoption. After doing some research, I discovered it is not an easy process and requires great financial resources and incomel. I began to wonder why it cost so much to adopt. This is not supposed to be business; it is act of kindness to humanity. We could save money for it; however, we faced an additional problem. When you are an American citizen, it is an easy process to get visa approval for your adoptive child. We are Palestinian, which means that we would have to go back and forth visiting a child or adoption agency in whatever country we were adopting.

Visiting Palestine as a tourist requires a visa that you cannot control. Sometimes they will give you only a few weeks or days to stay. This means if we decide to go live back home in Palestine, any child we adopt might not be able to return with us. It would require lawyers and thousands of dollars more to try to get a Palestinian passport for our adoptive child if he or she can even get one. Adopting a child is also a goal that I wanted to reach for a long time, even before getting married and dealing with infertility. I couldn't understand why there were children in orphanages suffering and missing parents when they could be with a family who could provide love, care, and better opportunities in life.

Foster care is another option, but social workers are usually working hard to reconnect their baby with biological parents, if possible. This means we could raise a child for a couple of years and then have someone knock on the door and tell us we have to give the child back to their biological parents. Even the idea of this was too painful to handle, so we skipped that option for now.

Growing up, becoming a mother was something that I always wanted to be. I wanted it very badly, since the first moments of our marriage. I was looking forward to pregnancy. When I started to have problems conceiving, medical conditions such as PCOS and endometriosis were the first two things that doctors identified. Some tests came back positive and others were negative. I was lost between doctors' clinics where everyone had different diagnoses and explanations. I needed to focus on making positive changes, improving myself, and learning all that I could.

Chapter 10

Continuing My Journey

I now had changed some habits in my life and felt better than ever. I was in better shape and I could tell my body and mind were responding positively to my new no-sugar, gluten-free, caffeine-free, and dairy-free diet. I also made mental changes and began to adopt a more positive attitude as I took responsibility for my life and my goals.

In the beginning, changing my diet, especially eliminating sugar, was hard. But I did it. Even with my new disciplined routine, I suddenly noticed I was eating a bit more. I even started craving sugar and had a hard time making myself eat healthy snacks. What was I doing wrong? I had to switch gears in my mind and tell myself that if I was able to eat healthy food, it would be OK if I had just a little bit of sugar. And guess what? That was all that I needed to continue eating well and reduce that bad habit automatically.

In addition to my dietary changes, I began exercising daily and drinking a lot more water. I added a few lemon pieces to my water to give me some variety. After a few months, I was doing great on this diet, I felt better, and my overall health seemed to improve.

It had been a few months into my new lifestyle when a random question came to me. Why I didn't get my menstrual cycle this month? Is my healthy lifestyle affecting it? I had heard that if women exercise more, it could affect their menstrual cycle, but I didn't know if that was it. I was a week late. Could it be my PCOS was getting worse? Deep inside me, I was not even thinking pregnancy, as I taught myself to stop expecting it. I decided to wait another week since I didn't have any symptoms. I continued with my new diet and lifestyle and distracted myself with work.

After two weeks, I was still late and decided to do a pregnancy test. I hadn't given up on our dream to have children, but I didn't want to get my hopes up. I told myself if I didn't get a positive result, there was always another chance later on.

I took the test and two lines appeared, though the second line was very, very faint. Was this a mistake? False positive result? Inaccurate test? Expired test?

I was probably just imagining it or maybe this test was wrong or too old. Should I tell Ali or wait? I was afraid to tell him and get him excited only to leave him disappointed and heartbroken again. I knew he was desperate for a baby. I decided to wait a couple of days and see. That seemed like a better idea if I could keep it inside me. All of the other times, I couldn't hold in my excitement and I told Ali right away. I did my best and kept this news to myself for two days.

When I took the test again, I saw two obvious lines. I swear it was darker than two days ago. *Now should I tell my husband or wait?* I wondered. But we hadn't done in vitro that month. I hadn't even visited my doctor in the last five weeks. I was confused, happy, scared, excited, and overwhelmed. It was a lot to process and keep to myself.

It was a regular night and I made a delicious dinner for both of us to enjoy. I enjoyed cooking every day and our meals were cleaner and healthier when I made meals from scratch. I wanted to wait until after dinner to tell my husband, but I couldn't wait any longer.

"Ali, I want to tell you something," I said. He looked at me and asked what was going on. I held the test with shaking hands and asked him if he could see both lines. His eyes opened wide as he looked up from the test to me.

"Yes! There are two lines!" he said, as the words escaped from his mouth.

Ali's reaction was unlike any I had seen in the videos that people post on social media where they start to scream, cry, or even laugh. I thought he was shocked or didn't believe it yet. We were both a little shocked, but cautiously optimistic.

Two hours later, I was surprised and disappointed to discover blood spotting. My quiet happiness turned to confusion and fear. I walked to the living room where Ali was watching a movie and my tears covered my cheeks. He was terrified and asked me what was going on. I told him and his eyes were teary, too. I wished I hadn't told Ali about the test. It was probably just another chemical pregnancy and my body was trying to get rid of it again. I wiped my tears away and managed to gather my strength and positivity back. I prayed to Allah to help me and I went to sleep. In the morning, I felt better. No more spotting or anything.

I thought it would be a good idea to call my doctor or send her a message the next day. My OB-GYN is more than a doctor to me Dr. Anwar Al-Kunani is my friend in this journey. She is like one of the family. I have known her for fourteen years and she had been trying her best to help us get pregnant. I was a hard, confusing, and challenging case for her. I think I was one of the oldest patients in her files. I sent her a picture of the positive pregnancy test.

She replied quickly with, "Did you do in vitro this month?" She probably thought I might have gone to another fertility clinic or done the IVF treatment overseas. I told her that we hadn't had any treatment, but I was scared because of the spotting. She told me to come in and get a blood test and we would see. The blood test also came back positive. However, the HCG level was very low, which was partly because my cycle was two weeks late. Right now, this was too weak of a sign to confirm a pregnancy this early. My doctor did not raise my hopes or even confirm pregnancy. It was a waiting game and we were praying that the following days would bring happiness to our little family.

Every two days, I repeated the blood test, and the levels kept increasing. Finally, the doctor felt confident enough with the results from the blood tests to confirm the pregnancy. We still had a long road to go to reach our goal of keeping this pregnancy and carrying it to full term.

Despite all this, I was pregnant without even doing any fertility treatments. Was this the miracle I had prayed for?

We took a test every two days to make sure my HCG level was increasing, and it was. After eight weeks, it was time to visit my doctor's office for an ultrasound to hear the baby's heartbeat. All this time, Ali didn't want to believe it, especially when I had no other signs of pregnancy like morning sickness. I was terrified, too. Why wasn't I vomiting like the women in the movies? I was not dizzy and I didn't have strange food cravings, except for a little sugar. All that time, I probably did twenty pregnancy tests and, of course, all of them were positive.

Walking to the clinic brought back a lot of memories. Oh, how many times had I walked away crying from that door and felt that no one really understood my pain? It was always such a crushing disappointment. But here I was, for the first time, walking into the clinic because I was already pregnant.

We were waiting in the room patiently, but we were still nervous. It seemed to take forever to start the ultrasound this time. Finally, the doctor came and my heart started to beat loud and fast. She looked at the screen and smiled. There it was: a tiny sac with a heartbeat.

We heard the baby's heartbeat for the first time. It was fantastic to hear someone else's heart beating inside me. We were two in one. Ali and I were both crying. I think this was the moment my husband finally *believed* it. We were officially pregnant but measuring six weeks of pregnancy instead of eight, because I ovulated late. That explained the late cycle and initial low levels of HCG on the tests. The sound of that baby's heartbeat took our breath away. My doctor seemed very serious as she focused on the screen, and that scared me. I asked if there was anything wrong. In the past, I had always heard the worst news at this point. Chemical pregnancy, blighted ovum, miscarriage. Was something wrong with the baby?

She looked at me and screamed, "You are having TWINS!" Still crying, a big smile crossed my face and I whispered, "Thank you, Allah."

My poor husband didn't say anything. He was in complete shock. Natural pregnancy with twins? After so many years of trying everything, we were now three in one. His reaction to the surprise was complete silence.

Now that the pregnancy was confirmed, and after we made it past eight weeks, I kept up with my healthy lifestyle and I started enjoying every minute of it. We announced the news to family and friends and their reactions were unbelievable, sweet, and loving. And, of course, the story itself amazed them. I think it took time for everyone to believe it was a natural pregnancy. They had been with us through all of our other highs and lows and everyone agreed this was a miracle.

Chapter 11

Staying Strong

Being pregnant with twins brought happiness to our small, growing family. Seeing them get bigger every two weeks on the ultrasound was amazing. But sometimes, sadness, fear, and frustration can walk through your dreams without permission or plans. I called them "challenges" instead of problems, and I love challenges. Going through a challenge can be frustrating, but for me, they made my dream and my road even more enjoyable and exciting.

My mother-in-law came to visit us. I was sitting on my living room sofa reading a book and took a moment to enjoy the smell of fresh bread filling the house from the loaf my mother-in-law was baking. Just then, something unexpected happened to spoil the cozy moment. I felt a strong contraction and had bleeding so heavy it soaked it through my pants to the couch. I was shocked and confused. Why was this happening? Was I having a miscarriage? Thankfully, I wasn't by myself at home and my mother-in-law rushed over to help.

We called Ali, who must have driven over the speed limit the whole way home. I was rushed to the emergency room. Losing my twins at 12 weeks was too painful to even think about. The bleeding was nonstop for an hour and took my breath away. It destroyed me. I searched my mind and remembered my lessons to stay strong and think positively. It might be hard to think positively in a negative situation, but I tried my best to apply everything I learned from my courses. I could do this. I did my best and prayed with a big smile and a full heart of faith to Allah to save my babies.

I knew that Allah was always there with his gracious power and he would bring the best for us and I trusted Him. I trust Him always. I did my work and just waited. After a couple of hours filled with tests and scans, the doctor came with an update. Our babies were fine and this was unrelated bleeding and not close to the babies. I was diagnosed with placenta previa, where the placenta covers the opening of the mother's cervix instead of being on the top of the babies.

To be honest, it wasn't easy to stay positive. I had to work through those natural emotions of fear and anxiety. It was especially hard as this wasn't the only occasion during the first trimester that I thought I could lose my babies. After this diagnosis, my doctor transferred me to a high-risk pregnancy team. I was smiling every time she looked in my eyes and said, "I am sorry, but you are a tough case."

I whispered to her, "You mean a *unique* case," and we both smiled.

In my situation, there was a combination of several issues that made this a high-risk pregnancy. First, they were dealing with placenta previa, which can cause bleeding throughout a pregnancy. I also had a short and weak cervix. The solution for a short cervix is a cerclage surgery where they put in some stitches to prevent late miscarriage or preterm birth. It was an easy step to do, but we were dealing with twins and they were afraid that the surgery stitches would cause my water to break.

We talked about the surgery to put in the stitches. In the tiny white room, the doctor took her glasses off and said, "You should be aware that you might lose both your babies or one of them." I looked back at her and told her not to worry about me. We would make it through.

And we did. For our weekly appointment at seventeen weeks, I was excited, since we would find out the gender of our babies. Ali wanted to know at that moment, but I was planning on having a gender reveal party so we would find out with our whole family. He couldn't wait and asked the ultrasound technician. She looked to me to see if I agreed to find out right away. I nodded my head "yes." Seeing Ali's happiness and excitement made me smile and I thought we should enjoy the moment together. Why wait for happiness? Let's take it.

We already knew that our babies were identical twins and they shared the same placenta, which was another thing that the doctors wanted to keep an eye on. They were worried that one of our babies would start to take more fluid than the other one and I was already starting to show signs of it. Twin A was swimming in more liquid volume than Twin B, but for now it was still within the acceptable range.

The ultrasound technician smiled and said, "Twin boys!"

I felt Ali's heart jump from his chest. I was over the moon, as it was the first time I saw a real reaction from Ali that was filled with both happiness and teary eyes. I don't remember seeing him that excited ever before in our married life. He gave me a big hug to celebrate and after the technician finished with all her measurements, she asked us to wait in the room to see the doctor. Why did I feel she was worried? Did she see something I didn't know about it? I tried to push my doubts aside to continue my moment of happiness with Ali.

Moments later, the doctor came into the room in a hurry and said that my cervix was very, very short and she thought I was already dilated. This meant I was possibly in labor. At seventeen weeks, the babies could not survive. She was correct. My cervix is short, and because of this, she recommended an emergency cerclage to try to save the babies if she could. We waited in the room while an operating room was being prepared to do the surgery within an hour.

I was sitting with Ali. He was worried but tried to act normally and told me silly jokes just to try to ease the situation for me. I was trying to laugh and I could see his mouth was moving, but I couldn't hear him talking. Things started to move faster around me, everything started to darken. The stark, white room suddenly became black. I whispered to Ali that I couldn't see anything, and that was the last thing I remembered.

I woke up after ten minutes in a different room with two doctors and a nurse trying to wake me up. I had completely fainted. It might have been how my body reacted to the fear and pain I was attempting to keep at bay. I felt better a few minutes later.

One hour later, I was in the operating room getting ready for the surgery. They used an epidural injection, the same injection they use for women in labor. The epidural was placed in my spine, which meant I had to stay as still as possible. The anesthesiologist was great about explaining everything. Within minutes, my legs started to go numb and felt like pieces of wood. I couldn't move them. They were heavy and I felt really weak.

In no time, the procedure was done, and everything seemed great. An hour later, I was feeling better. From that time, I was on bed rest for the duration of the pregnancy. Even with the cerclage, I needed to do whatever it took to prevent an early birth.

A few weeks later, I received a maternity dress that I ordered online for a photoshoot. I loved it! It was a long-sleeved maxi dress with sequins on the top part and flowy fabric on the bottom. I was hoping to get outside photos with a professional photographer. Unfortunately, I wasn't able to do the photoshoot I had dreamed about because of the stay-at-home and bed rest orders, and the photoshoot was postponed.

I was on strict bed rest for the rest of the pregnancy. No showers longer than two minutes and only twice a week. Our goal was to reach at least 30 weeks of pregnancy since the survival rate of the twins would be higher at that point. With my positive thinking, I turned what could have been boring, hard, and annoying bed rest into an enjoyable and productive time. In a few weeks, I finished my master's degree in learning and technology (through an online university) that I been working on from the previous year, watched my favorite movies, read a lot of books, and enrolled in self-development skill courses. I was blessed with my family. I will never forget their kindness and support as they fed me three meals a day, kept the house clean, and got everything I needed.

My dear husband was always there to provide love and support. At the 19-week appointment, everything seemed fine. We did the ultrasound and went home to find a lovely package waiting at our front door. It was my graduation gown and cap. Getting my master's degree was a dream that I achieved. I was hoping to attend the ceremony, but it wasn't possible.

Since I was not able to attend the ceremony, Ali had a surprise for me. He invited both of our families to our house to celebrate. I wore the maternity dress that I planned to wear in the photoshoots. My nieces helped me apply makeup and I looked beautiful. It had been a while since I had been all dressed up and fancy. With Ali's help and our hands entwined, I made it down to the family room. The whole house was decorated with balloons and banners. "You did it!" and "Congrats!" and many more. He did a great job bringing happiness to our house. All our families were there dancing to loud Arabic music, singing, and enjoying hot kanafeh for dessert. Kanafeh is a famous Middle Eastern dessert made of thin pastry, cheese, and hot sugar syrup.

I took a few pictures with the family and relaxed on the couch. It was a great hour with family, and I was so happy. Moments later, I started to feel dizzy, unbalanced, and tired. My mother noticed and asked how I was feeling. I whispered, "I am tired and want to go to bed."

My family members helped me upstairs, but I didn't make it to bed. I fainted on the stairs. I am glad they were holding me very tight. I woke up after twenty minutes to find myself in my bed, surrounded by my worried husband, terrified parents, and anxious brother. Everyone else was gone. The loud music was off and the family crowd had disappeared. They worried the party had been too much for me, but it hadn't. Their efforts had brought happiness and joy to my soul. I realized that I fainted, but this wasn't the first time and I thought it was related to low blood pressure. No need for doctors or ambulance. I felt absolutely fine within an hour.

I reached the 20-week mark and we were grateful for that. This was the first time I was showing a big belly, and I loved it. My babies were moving and kicking. It is amazing how you can feel another human inside you. With the two babies rolling around in my belly, a pregnancy pillow was a must. I rarely found a comfortable sleeping position.

My sister-in-law came to visit me and brought a delicious lunch with her. Suddenly, I started to have painful cramping that I couldn't hide. The cramping increased and I could feel pressure. My sister-in-law gently helped me get up from my bed.

I went to the bathroom and, again, I was bleeding. This time, I took a deep breath and managed not to let fear get to me. This had happened on and off, so I thought it could be normal for my unusual pregnancy. One hour later, the cramps were stronger and the bleeding was heavier. I called Ali, but he didn't answer and I figured he was a little bit busy at work or on another call. I texted him: "Ali I am having a little bit of cramping and a little bit of bleeding. Can you come to take me to the doctor?" He quickly arrived and we headed to the emergency room.

At the hospital, the monitor picked up a few contractions. They gave me more fluids and I was fine to go home the next day. My current high-risk team transferred me to a different high-risk team that specialized in cases with issues of identical twins sharing the same placenta. That was what they told me, but I worried that maybe they just wanted someone else to take responsibility for my unique case.

We had our first appointment with our new high-risk team, which was in a hospital about an hour from our house. The doctor did a great job explaining everything about our case. For the following weeks, we were monitoring the fluid in both babies. If the level kept increasing with Twin A and decreasing with Twin B, they would consider twin-to-twin transfusion surgery. I had never heard of it and didn't know of anyone who had gone through that surgery.

Let me be honest. I was scared and I tried to build my positive energy up for that day, but I failed. This possibility was too overwhelming and scary. However, I did understand that any human can face a challenge and have moments of failure and doubt. I allowed myself a few hours to be sad and frightened, and I was able to regain my positivity to face those very challenging days. You cannot reach a dream without challenges. They are always a part of any goal or dream.

Our doctor was one of the most amazing doctors I have ever met. He had an incredible level of education and experience, but he was also a compassionate human being. My team decided I should stay in the hospital for a couple of weeks so they could do a daily ultrasound to measure the fluid level for each baby. I didn't mind the constant supervision and seeing my babies daily on the ultrasound screen was remarkable. I distracted myself by watching videos and reading books to support my need for motivation.

I will never forget that moment when the doctor told me that surgery was a must and he would try his best to send one baby home as I was only twenty three week pregnant. *What? I am pregnant with twins! What do you mean "one baby" and not two?*

He told me, "I will be honest with you, this surgery is very risky, especially with the short cervix. We may lose one baby or two, but I will try my best to save you."

I understand that patients should be informed and know what is going on with their case but, to be honest, this felt like too much information. This was a serious life or death situation. I could lose one baby, both of them or all three of us could die. I flipped the statement in my head and told myself that he will save the babies and I will be just fine. I had to focus on that thought. The alternative was too scary.

I had been through a lot of challenges. I could do this. It was just a surgery; a small surgery that would last three hours. I got my motivation and hopes up. What else could I do? Sit around crying? No, I wasn't going to cry. They told me that babies at that age feel their mother's emotional states and I didn't want the twins to feel that I was crying, stressed, or feeling sad. *We will be fine*. I wrapped my hands around my belly to comfort my babies.

"Hang in there, boys. Mama loves you," I whispered to them.

Chapter 12

Being Fearless

You might be wondering at this point and think I was just lying to myself, but I wasn't. The doctors were just making predictions. The worst outcome didn't have to be my reality. It might happen and it might not. Why should I think the worst and scare myself? With fear, our immune system is lowered, our heartbeat increases, and we still have no power to change the outcomes.

I always wondered why children tolerated surgeries better than adults, and I think it is the fear factor. Imagine a soldier who is scared in a battle. It's healthy to have some fear, but if that soldier lets fear overtake them, will they win or survive? I don't think so.

As I write this, we are dealing with COVID-19 crisis and everyone is terrified. In our state, Illinois, the numbers are scary and increasing every day. I did have a moment that I was worried about my family members, especially my parents, but for now, I almost forget about it. We do what is recommended to prevent spreading the virus. We are staying home, washing our hands frequently, eating healthy foods to support the immune system, and washing and sanitizing everything we purchase.

Like everything else in life, I try to take the positive side. During this pandemic, we are home, spending time with family, reading more, relaxing, cooking healthy new recipes, organizing our home, and deep cleaning. I can call an old friend and chat with them, take an online course, and many more things. I now have more appreciation for our normal, regular days. We used to complain about those regular days of stress, annoyances, or boredom. Now we are just hoping that the days that we were bored or complaining about will come back.

Back in the operating room, I was prepped for the twin-to-twin transfusion surgery. In an effort to remain positive and fearless, I told myself I would be safe with my boys, no matter what. Right before they gave me general anesthesia, a doctor approached and asked me if I had blood problems. I told him I did faint a couple of times during the pregnancy, but I thought it was low blood pressure. They decided I needed to have a blood transfusion before they started because I was in a dangerous anemic state. This blood transfusion was a must before the surgery.

The nurses looked worried. Everyone was very sympathetic since they knew about my struggle to get pregnant. I started to make silly jokes and we all laughed a little. I did have moments of fear sneaking into my heart, but I can say I managed to stay 80 percent positive most of the time. The last thing I remember before the sedation was moving my hand toward my belly and praying that Allah will protect the twins.

Hours passed and I woke up touching my stomach to make sure I was still pregnant. I could still feel my big pregnant belly. I asked my beautiful nurse if I was still pregnant and she answered, "Yes. With both babies." I was so happy and I told her to swear that she was telling the truth! We both laughed and I hugged her.

I don't know if it was the reaction to anesthesia or just the love that my heart holds for nurses after every surgery, but I always hug the nurse who is taking care of me. They are the angels of love and mercy on earth. I appreciate their work in caring for others.

The best way I know to fight fear is think to positively, imagine the best, and exchange fear for gratitude. Things could always be worse, so I thank Allah for that and smile, laugh, and make myself and those around me happy.

Two days after the surgery and it was Ramadan. Everyone was happy, fasting and gathering at night together to break their fast with delicious food and sweets. By this point, things looked great. The fluid volumes were now equal and the surgery was a big success. I asked Ali to go home and sleep there that night. I felt good and there was no need to stay in the hospital with me. Our home was an hour away and I wanted him to get some good rest. He had been sleeping on the hospital couch for days.

That night after Ali left, I read a couple of pages of the holy Quran, watched a short movie, and was ready to sleep. Monitors were on 24 hours a day to make sure my babies were doing well. They were poking and prodding me, and the beeping machines were bothering me, but I would handle anything for the sake of my twins. Around two in the morning, the door flew open violently, someone turned on all the lights, and four nurses came running in. One of them was calling and saying something about C-section, the others grabbed me quickly and flipped me to my left side, I was terrified. I asked what was going on, but they didn't answer. They were busy doing their work. It was only a couple of minutes, but it felt like an hour. Finally, one of them told me that Twin B's heartbeat was dropping, and they were going to do an emergency C-section.

I needed to let my husband know.

The nurses were busy looking and watching the beeping screen and a doctor came running in. I managed to grab my cell phone and called Ali. I imagined that he probably had a panic attack from my call, hearing the fear in my voice and C-section news. Five minutes later, everything was back to normal and Twin B's heartbeat was going strong again. I called my husband to tell him everything was fine, and he was thrilled to hear that. The doctors didn't know the reason for it, but thought the baby was holding tight to his umbilical cord. There was never a dull moment for me and the babies.

Time kept marching on and three weeks in the hospital had passed. I was now twenty five weeks along in our pregnancy. I missed my house a lot. Doctors did their rounds and the surgery was a great success. Soon,

I could leave the hospital and everything seemed good. I was ready to go home and follow up with my OB-GYN for the rest of my pregnancy. Ali helped me to get organized and ready for the long drive home during rush hour traffic.

On the way home, my brother called to check on me. He invited us to his house for a big family dinner that night. It would be such a boost to see all of them. I almost said "no" because I just wanted to go home, but his house was easy to get to and I did miss my family. Spending a couple of hours with them would be great. Slowly, I got out of the car and they helped me over to the comfy couch. I wanted to take a shower. It had been a long week after the surgery and I seriously needed one. I took a quick shower at my brother's house while sitting on a chair. It did the trick, and I was once again clean and fresh.

I was sitting on the couch in my comfortable pajamas watching TV with my family when I started to feel pressure and contractions. My contractions were hard and painful. In the beginning, I tried to hide it and thought it could be random cramping, so I took one pain pill. Politely, I asked for help to go to sleep in the bedroom. I took a short nap, but my contractions came back.

I started to track them and didn't tell anyone. I tried to avoid worrying everyone around me. The contractions were now every eight minutes. *What should I do? I need to go back to the hospital,* I told myself. I decided to wait until dinner was done and let Ali take me back. I now felt the pain was manageable. Ali came to hold my hand and helped me reach the car to go home. I was excited to return to my own space.

Standing up slowly, I felt a huge splash of warm liquid all over my pants. It only took seconds and the floor was covered with blood. I could see the shocked faces around me looking at each other. I didn't say a word. I was too puzzled to say anything.

Ali acted fast and called the doctor at home. He gave Ali his private number and told him to call him anytime if we needed anything. Did I mention he is the most human doctor out there? He assessed the situation quickly and told Ali to take me back to the labor and delivery suite as soon as possible.

Chapter 13

Getting Ready

It was a long ride back to the hospital and I needed a blanket to cover myself in order to absorb all of the moisture as it felt like I was still bleeding heavily. Ali was driving so fast that I wished the police were there to stop us.

"Ali, calm down, honey. I feel much better," I said, trying to talk him down from his panic.

The road was very dark. Was it the road or were my eyes starting to go dark? I thought I would faint soon. Ali noticed my condition and started to talk to me to grab my attention and keep me awake. His voice was shaking and scared. I couldn't understand what he was saying.

Once we arrived at the hospital, we reached the nurse's station and they hurried me into a room. We rushed to the bathroom to clean me up after all of the blood.

"Will I lose my babies?" I asked.

"I don't know, sweetheart," replied the nurse.

This time it was seriously dangerous. I have been having contractions every three minutes over the last couple of hours. I was tired. I mean exhausted! Once they checked me, I was relieved to discover that my cervix was at four centimeters dilated, even with the stitches still attached. I tried to keep the fear at bay, but I understood my situation. I was in labor. But I was only 25 weeks pregnant.

This would take a strong heart and I had no choice but to go with the flow and know that whatever was going to happen would happen. But for now, *Can I cry for five minutes? I mean, ten minutes?* I had my full ten minutes of hard crying. The kind of crying where my shoulders shook hard with every breath. This was the best way to get all the negative feelings out of my body. Ten minutes later, I felt better and more ready to face the dire situation.

Our hospital room was filled with doctors and nurses. Tests and ultrasound scans showed that my babies were doing well. However, Twin A's water had broken. The plan was to keep monitoring 24/7. We were buying time. A day or even a few hours would help. The room I was in was a labor and delivery suite ready with equipment, and there were two baby beds standing by for any emergencies.

The sight of those beds inspired mixed feelings. I was happy to see two cribs waiting for my boys and excited to be able to meet them. But we were supposed to meet them in August, not in May! *Did you miss Mommy so much that you broke your water?* I teased the little one most at risk inside me.

The neonatal intensive care unit (NICU) staff kept coming back and forth to explain the possibility of my babies surviving. They mentioned every possible issue or problem that we could face. To be honest, I wasn't paying close attention and didn't take them seriously. I understood the situation, but I believe in Allah and I could feel it down in my heart. I would not expect anything. I would go with the flow. I didn't have the power or health to stand against this strong storm on my own. I would trust in Allah as I had in the past.

Several medications, such as Terbutaline, were given to try to stop the contractions. Everything failed. The bleeding was nonstop and the painful contractions came every three minutes. I tried my best to manage my pain by breathing deeply. Things were getting serious and the pain was so bad that I started to scream.

A new nurse came in and introduced herself. This was the first time I really felt I had a nurse who was careless, unprofessional, and not very attentive. Even though she was supposed to be by me all the time, she was in a different world. I think she was having a bad day. I was in a busy intensive care unit for pregnant women. I appreciated all of their hard work, but after seeing the attitude of that new nurse, I didn't expect much from them, and if I needed anything that I could do by myself, I didn't want to call them.

Ali was also next to me and he was very supportive, providing anything I needed. However, there are things like medication and painkillers that only the nurses can administer. Late in the evening, Ali was tired and fell asleep on the couch.

Two long days passed filled with contractions and bleeding. I asked the nurse if she could get me a painkiller to ease my pain and hopefully let me take a nap. She said "yes," but didn't bring me anything. Instead she came back with new monitor strips to try to track the babies' heartbeats. For two days, they were having a tough time trying to capture the babies' heartbeats and track them on the monitor..

My babies were very active. She made many attempts to find the heartbeats but she couldn't. After fifteen minutes of pain inflicted by her attempts at squeezing my belly, I asked her to stop and call the doctor. In the past, when they have a hard time, they usually bring out a tiny ultrasound to find the heartbeats to avoid the pain and struggle. She refused and said that she had "magic hands" that no other nurse had. I didn't say a word. Another ten minutes of her trying to painfully locate the heartbeats and I had finally had enough.

"I am done! Please at least grab some pain medicine and then you can continue," I said firmly.

"Mama, you need to understand that I know my job," she replied.

"Wait, what? I am the one who is suffering and my bleeding is getting heavier from all your squeezing! Stop! Go get the doctor!"

Thankfully, this time she did stop and my lovely on-call doctor came running in to discover that my bleeding was getting worse, and she called another doctor to join her. The doctor arrived in a rush and told me that they would pull the cerclage stitches and see if I could handle it for another few hours before the babies were delivered. Twin A's head was down, but Twin B was breech, so a C-section was a must. The anesthesiologist was present for the epidural injection to take the stitches out. I didn't even feel the needle poke my skin. I think I had become so used to the pain that a little needle was nothing at that point.

The doctor whispered to my husband that the bleeding was some of the worst he had seen in his life and they needed to save me, the mother. Despite his attempts to be discreet, I heard it very clearly.

I said, "No, please. Doctor, wait! I don't want to deliver now. The time is important. I can handle it."

He looked at me with his eyes wide in disbelief. He said, "I am sorry, but I have to save you. If you keep bleeding like this another hour, your life is in danger." He looked to his nurse and ordered the emergency C-section.

It was a scary moment for us. Ali hugged me and I cried loudly from deep in my lungs. Ali gazed into my eyes and said, "Look at me. You are going to be fine. Our boys will make it. Relax, and let's enjoy these moments. In the end, it is the birth of our boys."

He was absolutely right. This was the birth of our boys. I started to breathe normally and was amazed at how fast they transported me to the operating room. It only took a couple of minutes and Ali joined me, wearing his mask and sterile hospital outfit. He looked like a doctor. I mean, a very handsome doctor.

Chapter 14

The Big Day

In the operating room, there were almost 30 doctors, nurses, and medical staff. I had never seen anything like the two baby beds that were there. They were small units that closed up and had a lot of wires and machinery. The epidural was given, intravenous meds and fluids were connected, and a big drape was hung to make sure we weren't seeing any of the procedures and to give the doctors a more focused surgical field. I am glad that they cover everything. I don't think many women could handle to seeing their stomach cut wide open.

They cleaned my belly and were ready to open me up. There was a nurse standing next to me to give all of the updates. I was feeling fine overall; no real pain throughout the procedure, just a little bit of pressure when they pulled my babies out. I am forever grateful for modern medicine that makes surgeries pain-free. They shouted "Hi!" and baby Rawhi was out, crying in a very soft voice that made my heart melt and my eyes drop happy tears. They didn't show him to me because he needed oxygen support immediately. I was wondering what he looked like. Did he resemble me or his dad?

His crying made me cry more. They were tears of joy and concern. Ali was crying, too, and holding my hand. We were parents. We had made it. Finally, we were a Mom and a Dad. It was an amazing moment. We had been waiting for this for a very long time; long, long years filled with failure and disappointment. A good part of our marriage was related to infertility, but with wisdom and work we were able to stay together and become even stronger and feel more love than ever. I think in that time of trial we discovered how important and worthy our life together was. Those fourteen years played in a short movie in front of my eyes. All the failure, tears, and struggle vanished with Rawhi crying and our welcoming him to the world.

Another "Hi!" and the birth of Yaseen brought me to the reality that was happening in the operating room. I was waiting to hear his voice, too. But I didn't. I didn't hear Yaseen crying. A sudden silence fell over the team.

Ali was trying his best to comfort me and moving to sneak a look behind the big divider to check in on baby Yaseen. I looked at my husband with questioning in my eyes.

"Ali, I didn't hear Yaseen crying. Did you hear him?" I asked.

I hoped he told me he did, But he shook his head "no." My heart dropped.

"Is my baby fine?" I asked. No one answered.

I managed to stay calm and think positive. I asked one more time and they finally told us that he came out a little blue and was having a hard time taking a breath, but he was fine now and breathing. I took a deep breath, too. A smile formed on my face as we were all now alive and breathing together.

The whole procedure was done within 45 minutes. The doctor left and nurses took over to close the stiches. I saw the two mini cribs wheel past my bed and through the doors. I tried my best to see them, but I wasn't successful. I was left still wondering what they looked like. One thing was for sure, I knew they were handsome.

Within an hour, the hospital waiting room was filled with our families who were both terrified and excited. Many emotions were swirling around the room; all feelings of happiness and concern for our babies' overall health. How wonderful to have family and friends around us! They are truly a blessing.

I had been given two units of a blood transfusion to help boost my body and recover all the lost blood, which helped. But I was now in the recovery room dealing with epidural side effects. Shaking hands and overall body pain lasted for two hours. I felt my bones were broken, and I was tired, exhausted, and concerned about my babies (even though I tried my best not to worry).

Ali swore to me that our boys were doing well. They weighed one pound and four ounces each. He showed me pictures and videos. I was not allowed to get out of bed to go and see my babies. Around midnight, I had a very bad reaction to morphine that caused me to be awake all night with an itchy face and body. I think I was allergic to it, but never knew before then. I was awake all night and managed to pump breast milk three times. When the nurse came and asked me to rest and take care of myself, I told her about the itchiness and reaction to the medication and she switched it to another one. I think the excitement and worry about my babies made the sleep hide from my eyes. I couldn't wait until morning to go and see them.

May 9th was the best day of my life as I officially became a Mommy. What a beautiful Mother's Day gift for that year.

Finally, morning arrived. The beautiful sunrise added shine to my life and boosted my spirits as I tried to get out of bed for the first time. My abdomen was sore and swollen and I couldn't move my body alone. I had never experienced pain like I was experiencing in that moment, but I loved it because the pain and joy would forever remind me of my motherhood journey. With help and support from both my nurse and Ali, I managed to reach my wheelchair. Healing is a process, and it was amazing to see and feel how the human body can heal. We are amazing creations. I could handle pain and I knew I would be feel great again in a few days as my body worked to heal itself.

Ali and I traveled through the hospital hallways and my heart was beating fast like it did on our first date. This was the first time meeting our boys. How I could not be excited? I entered the NICU, washed my hands up to the elbow, signed the papers, and was led to my boys' room.

The nurse pointed to Rawhi and said that he was Twin A. To be honest, I didn't see much of him. What I did see was a small incubator with a small crib, and inside that was a very tiny human covered with wires, breathing tubes, and a piece of fabric over his eyes. I took five minutes of silence to try to understand the sight. In the pictures that Ali showed me, they seemed bigger, longer, and healthier. My heart jumped from my chest. It was love at the first sight. The nurse opened the small window and I put my hand inside to touch his hand. He held on to my finger. *He knows me! I am his Mama,* I thought.

We moved to Yaseen's crib and he was identical to Rawhi. He even wrapped his little hand around my finger. I was crying and couldn't stop. I was overjoyed to call these tiny humans my sons. Double the cuteness, double the love. And most of all, double the blessings.

They were so tiny, only one pound, four ounces each. Their skin, face, and body was different from any newborn I had known. They were here and we were so happy.

It was a whole different world behind the NICU doors. There are worried and exhausted faces all around and parents are holding their baby's tiny hands just as we did. Some babies were bigger than mine. We were at Pod A for the tiny special care unit. I'm not in the medical field and English is my second language, so it was sometimes hard to understand all the medical terms they used. I made sure to smile at everyone each time I walked through the aisle. I hoped that my smile would make them smile, too, and let the other parents know they were not alone.

Every day a doctor came around and talked to us about our babies' progress. After they finished their daily updates, I always asked them if the babies were OK overall. They said, "Yes, but they need special attention for a long time." Of course, they were born at 25 weeks and they required extra care. We would support them as much as we could to help them fight and grow bigger and stronger.

In the NICU, we had good days and very tough ones, as the nurses described them every time I called to check in. I believe they were all good days as even the tough days were part of their growth. Since day one, they told us that the first two weeks were very critical. Two weeks in, and Rawhi was sicker than Yaseen. I visited them daily and spent hours by their sides, speaking words of love and providing "kangaroo holding" for them. We were then, as we are now, so much in love.

Chapter 15

Survival

On May 21st, I visited our boys as usual. Up until that point they hadn't opened their eyes yet. With the help of four nurses, they handed me Yaseen to hold him and provide skin-to-skin contact and love. He was getting cozy between my arms. I lost myself in that moment and I was up over the clouds when Yaseen opened his eyes for the first time. On May 21st, Ali and I visited our boys as usual."
    looked at him with love and surprise. I was wondering if he was seeing me! Maybe not, but for sure he was feeling safe and loved with his Mama. It was one of the best days, seeing his tiny eyes open. Welcome to your new world, Sweetheart.
    The next day, I got a random call from my husband to get ready to go visit our twins in the NICU. They were two weeks old at this point. This was strange because we were already going to visit the boys at a scheduled time each day. The sound of his shaking voice was enough to get me worried. I got ready and waited for him. When I climbed into the car I realized he was crying, and at that moment my heart stopped.

"Talk to me. What is going on?" I asked. He told me that he had received a call from the NICU and the doctor informed him that Yaseen was not doing well.

"OK," I replied. "You know how it is in the NICU. We have tough days." I had called two hours ago and the nurse told me he was doing find and they were just waiting to do an x-ray for him. Yaseen was showing symptoms of necrotizing enterocolitis, known as NEC, which was very hard for me to understand and I had to use Google Translate to read about it. It is an inflammation of the intestines which can cause holes or damage and allow bacteria to infect the baby. The trip took 40 minutes, but it felt like three hours.

We got another phone call while we were on the road to let us know that Yaseen needed emergency surgery as soon as possible. We gave permission for the doctors to start. Then, just as we pulled into the parking lot, there was another phone call to ask where we were. This call confused me because Yaseen had been in surgery for only fifteen minutes or so and they were already calling to check on us. We were afraid that there might be something wrong that they couldn't say on the phone.

The doctors were waiting for us as we entered the hospital. That was not a good sign and fear flooded my heart. I asked where Yaseen was, and the doctor took us to a corner to talk to us first. He was having a hard time speaking, but he managed to put his words together and told us he was sorry, but Yaseen wasn't going to make it and would likely pass away within two hours.

Everything around me started to move quickly. I was dizzy. I hurried to the NICU pod where Rawhi was sleeping in his bed, but Yaseen's bed was missing. They showed us the emergency operating room they used in the same NICU unit. This was a nightmare and I wanted Ali to shake me and wake me up in a few seconds, but he didn't. He couldn't It wasn't a bad dream. It was real life. Within an hour, all our family were next to us. I had never heard Ali crying so loudly and deeply, and I never imagined the pain of saying goodbye to our son.

I took the blanket he was covered with, even though there was still some blood on it. Losing your baby is one of the most devastating things any human can face. I felt that everything was frozen around me. I couldn't feel my legs. I think my soul traveled to somewhere else. The reality hit me hard this time. There was no positive scenario I could create or think of to make this better. I couldn't just think positively or smile this away. We entered the small operating room in the NICU unit and my baby Yaseen was lying in that bed, covered with blood. They opened his stomach to cut out the infected intestine, but there was nothing they could save or remove.

I stood behind the door waiting for a miracle to happen. *But what miracle is there? He is passing away. Wake up and deal with it*, I told myself. They opened the door and everyone was teary, maybe from hearing my loud cries. They told me I could hold him and we could choose to take our baby off of life support. I refused. I told them to just leave it to help him to survive. I held his tiny body in my hands and kissed him more than any time before. I just hugged and kissed him for two hours.

Ali was broken. He was crying like I had never seen him cry before. The machines started to beep and baby Yaseen's hands and legs began to freeze and stiffen. The doctors rushed in and asked me if I agreed to have them do CPR. I looked at their faces. One doctor told me his stomach is open and CPR would break his ribs. Next to me, my brother whispered, "Don't do it. Let him pass peacefully."

In a few moments, Yaseen was gone.

Yaseen's soul went up to heaven as I held him in my arms. We were crushed. No. That's not even a strong enough word to describe the pain. I don't think there are words in any language to equal the anguish that we felt. Everyone, including the medical staff, was in tears. My story with infertility touched them deeply in the heart. Mine was not a story they wanted to hear every day. They used to call them miracle twins! My crying was loud, very loud, that shaded a sadness all over the NICU. Parents, staff, and everyone around looked at us with teary eyes. I felt that this pain would never end. My life stopped and my heart was broken. I actually felt as if my heart was bleeding.

An hour later, people from the funeral service were there to pick him up. It was hard to let him go alone with them, but Rawhi was still there, fighting for his life, and leaving him alone was not an option. Looking at both rooms in front of me, I realized in one room, Yaseen was going with the funeral service people, and in the next room, Rawhi was fighting for his life. *Where should I go? I can't just hand Yaseen over to them and I can't leave Rawhi?* It was an agonizing decision.

I asked to spend my time with Yaseen and I hugged him very tight, close to my heart for hours. I kissed every inch of his one-pound body. *I wish I could give you my life to live!* As I held him, my C-section began to hurt like the first day. I could barely move and asked for a strong pain killer to manage it. Time went by too fast and soon it was time for them to take Yaseen. My son needed to go to his next life.

With the help of family, I walked slowly through the hallway—broken—to reach my Rawhi's crib. I sat next to his bed, holding his hand. I told him to fight as much as he could. I knew his tiny soul could feel the loss of his twin brother and I wanted to comfort him, even though I knew there were no words for what we were feeling in that moment. Our boys were together for six months in a tiny place sharing food from the same placenta, kicking each other sometimes, and laying on top of each other most of the time. And now one of them was gone from this earth.

It had only been two weeks since the twins were born, and my body and C-section were hurting badly from all that crying and pressure. After a while, I went home to rest, as my family and Ali forced me to do. I couldn't argue more because I didn't even have the power to say anything. I was extremely exhausted.

In the Muslim religion, the funeral tradition is to bury the loved one as soon as possible. Yaseen's funeral service was on the second day after his passing. Seeing him in that small box terrified me. It made his death real and final. Burying a loved one is one of the most painful feelings that you can face, but burying a child brings unimaginable grief. I survive by speaking to Yaseen and keeping him in my mind and heart. *I miss you a lot, Sweetheart. Not one day passes without me thinking of you and remembering you opening your tiny eyes and feeling your heart beating next to mine.*

As I write this, it was almost a year ago, but it feels like yesterday. Yaseen's soul went up to heaven, to a better place, and he is looking at us with his smile that I didn't have the chance to see. I had three days of nonstop crying because once the shock and numbness wore off, I was aware of what I was going through. I had to let all that sadness out. It is human nature to feel sad about losing a beloved one, especially a baby. When Prophet Mohammed lost his baby son, Ibrahim, he said, "Indeed, the eyes shed tears and the heart is grieved and we don't say except what pleases our lord. And indeed, over your departures, O Ibrahim, we are grieved."

There must be some hidden wisdom or reason for losing Yaseen, but I wasn't able to see it in that moment. After three days, I was ready to go back, hold my head up, and muster all the strength I had to give Rawhi the support he needed to fight and survive. He was still in critical condition. Actually, they told us since day one that Rawhi was much sicker than Yaseen. But doctors are only human, and although they told us all of the possibilities, they can't predict the future.

July 1st came. It was our anniversary! Since it was our first anniversary as parents, we wanted to go celebrate next to Rawhi, as we did every day. What could be more special than spending this day next to our son? Rawhi was getting bigger every day. He was now 36 weeks old. While we were prepared to bask in the celebration the day brought, he had other plans and decided to celebrate our anniversary in his own way.

While standing there next to his crib, his nurse was getting ready to take his temperature. The machine started to beep, his lips turned blue, and doctors rushed into the room. Rawhi had stopped breathing and his heart stopped for a few seconds.

I stood there in the hallway in the same spot where the doctor had announced the loss of Yaseen. I closed my eyes, took deep breaths, and raised my hand to the sky to pray to Allah. *Please save him, be next to him.* I found myself sitting on the floor just watching from afar. I kept running positive thoughts through my head. Moments later, the machine stopped beeping and everything returned back to normal. What happened? No one really knew. Maybe he just got so excited about our anniversary and wanted to surprise us? Maybe he was joking? *Sorry, son, but I didn't like your joke!*

Days passed in the NICU and my Rawhi was getting stronger and healthier. He had been there for five full months and he weighed nine pounds, however, Rawhi was still on all kinds of life support. He did have another few episodes where his heart almost stopped, but he is a fighter and God blessed him.

Rawhi was moved from one room to another as his health improved, and we began preparing for his graduation from the NICU. All kinds of therapies and medications were provided. We agreed to keep Rawhi's health records private and only for him. It is his story, and he is the only one who can talk about it and decide when the time is right to share it or not. He spent 147 days behind closed doors, in the NICU, and each day was different than the next. Days full of tears, pain, smiles, and growing stronger.

Walking through the NICU, you will see moms and dads crying, and it will break your heart. I had a conversation with a mother who had a story that was similar to mine. One of her twins had been through eight surgeries and would need many more. It was very painful to see her child suffering from pain. In that moment, I thanked God. Losing Yaseen was very tough on me, but he is now in a better place where he is happy and safe, and at least he is not suffering. Everything happens for a reason, even if that reason is hidden during that moment. Not one day passes without remembering my boy, but now I can smile because he is not suffering. His little soul is flying peacefully.

Rawhi continues to grow and thrive. He is a healthy baby and the joy of our lives. We will always remember the care and kindness shown to us by medical professionals and our families. It may have taken fourteen years for Rawhi and Yaseen to arrive, but the struggle and the pain was worth all of the joy and love that we feel. We finally have our family.

Section Two

PERSONAL GROWTH

Introduction

When I started writing this book, I wasn't sure if it was a memoir or a self-help book. I wanted to share my story and give hope and encouragement to other people struggling with infertility. I also wanted to share the changes and improvements that I made in my health, my mind, and my attitude during this period and beyond. I want to share some of the things I learned to help anyone who is chasing their dreams or working toward accomplishing a goal. I think it is the teacher in me that wants to help others.

This section details some of the things and changes that had a tremendous impact on my life. I hope that you can find something here that speaks to you and gives you the courage to stay on your own path of believing in yourself and achieving any goal you set your mind to accomplishing.

Chapter 16

Time Management and Organization

Time Management

One of the biggest changes I made to my lifestyle was improving my time management. If you have a dream, your busy lifestyle can make it a challenge to reach it. Unless you take control of your schedule and your time, you will continue to feel like there are not enough hours in the day to get everything done. Time management is an important life skill that you can learn and apply to every part of your life.

I was trapped in that mindset, too. I was complaining about how fast my days went by and I never had extra time for other projects or goals. Between my job as an online seller, family time, household responsibilities, and studying for my master's degree, time just flew by. By the end of the day, I didn't have the power or energy to do anything and I would just lie on the couch and then go to bed. Weekends were spent deep cleaning around the house, grocery shopping, and preparing for the new week. Sunday was Ali's day off and this became the only day to spend time together and meet up with our extended families for gatherings or just to enjoy visiting with each other.

Creating a schedule is one of the first things to consider in order to improve your time management. I wrote my schedule based on my job and family commitments. By looking at your schedule on paper (or on a computer or a phone), you will discover that you do have some extra time built in to do other things. I give myself a Task List every day, making allowances for some flexibility or last-minute changes. Then I list those tasks in order of priority and focus first on the most important must-do tasks. Doing this means you will feel a great sense of accomplishment as you check each completed task off your list. You will also realize how much time you were spending on non-productive things like watching TV or playing games on your phone. You can build in time for these fun activities, but don't let them take over your entire day and stop your progress.

Stick to your schedule for at least twenty days, and after that, it will become a habit that is easy to follow. Having a routine will not only help you manage your time better, but it will help your family, especially children, have a predictable routine. Every night at bedtime, I write my tasks for the following day in order, starting with the most important to the least. I also take tasks that I didn't complete and move them to the next day. The tasks that you didn't get to will be a higher priority the next day.

I use an app that I downloaded to my phone to help me stay organized and it does make my day much easier to follow. In my daily routine, I created my Task List to include physical exercise, meditation, reading, and working online in my shop.

I had several reasons for leaving teaching, some of them related to the complicated schedules of our IVF treatments. When I left teaching, I couldn't start the semester because I was overseas to do in vitro, and I was looking for a better opportunity with flexible hours. I switched to being a substitute teacher in my school district and started my online shop selling women's apparel. This gave me flexible hours and better income.

Even with a schedule where I could set my own hours, and wake up whenever I wished, I started waking up earlier. Just starting my day one hour earlier doubled the productivity in my day. Having that one hour of no distractions, kids, phone, or emails is really like four hours of trying to get things with the whole household awake and the morning in full swing. Just one hour first thing in the morning makes a huge difference.

I also give myself a firm bedtime and avoid staying up late. I am usually in bed by 10:30 p.m. at the latest and wake up by 6:00 a.m. every day. This habit helps me stick to this routine every day at the same time, no matter if it is on the weekend or a regular day. I have been amazed at the quality of sleep I got when I adopted a firm bedtime. Before, I usually woke up tired. Now I wake up full of energy. In the first couple of days, I would go to bed by 10:00 p.m. and stay awake for an hour before finally falling asleep, but now I fall asleep easily. I think it is because I have more control over finishing tasks and have less worry and stress.

One final tip: Invest in a good mattress. We spend a lot of money for new clothes, eating at restaurants, and buying new cars but we spend at least eight hours of our day in bed and often skimp on the cost of a mattress. You deserve a comfortable mattress that will help you feel refreshed. Don't wake up with aches and pains from an uncomfortable mattress.

Get Organized

There are several reasons why you should be organized. Staying organized saves time. If your goal involves a lot of steps and appointments, like mine did, you will have to be on top of things and stay organized. For instance, if you plan on what you will wear and lay your clothes out the night before, you can probably cut out 30 minutes in the morning searching for the complete outfit to wear. Imagine how much time you could save by making this one change.

Doing this with your children will also save a lot of time looking. How many mornings have you wasted time looking for that one pair of shoes that your kid insists on wearing? Taking a few minutes every evening to plan your child's outfit and get their schoolwork organized will save you a lot of aggravation and time the next day. Plus, the more you instill these habits in your children, the more pleasant your household will be and the more successful they will be in the future. No more rushed mornings of trying to find a backpack or a favorite shirt.

Being organized will save you money. Have you ever rushed to the store to purchase just a few things needed and ended up with a full cart? It seems like the story of my life! And, of course, I buy the extra stuff because I don't remember if we have some at home or because I don't want to run out of it. By having a more organized pantry and having a detailed shopping list, you will save money.

Being organized will reduce your stress level. The process of cleaning, organizing, and getting rid of extra stuff that we didn't use really gave me true peace of mind and less stress. For a regular person like me, it was not an easy process. I usually care about keeping the house clean, but I wasn't paying attention to how much organizing would have a great impact on our life.

Now everything has a place and there are no excuses for throwing stuff all around the house, no matter how much I am tired or in a hurry. How does that help me to reach my goal? Not searching for lost keys or having dirty laundry all over the house allowed me more free time to do research and focus on my goals and dreams. In that additional time, I can prepare healthy clean meals to ensure that we are maintaining a healthy diet and encourage us as a family to stay away from fast food and takeout meals. Can you see how doing this also saves money?

Being organized will give you more free time. For me, I have more time to take a walk around the neighborhood, which improves my overall physical health and reduces my stress level. I have more time for meditation. During meditation, I like having essential oils, candles, or just that clean smell of a peaceful and welcoming house that sneaks into your nose and impacts the meditation experience. Whether you make quiet time for prayer or meditation, you deserve this time every day.

This all sounds great, but what if you are overwhelmed and don't know where to start?

I use a method with a 30-minute timer. Before going to bed, set a 30-minute timer and do the following: Take the trash out, collect any toys or any objects on the floor, wash any dishes or load and start the dishwasher, and then go to bed. In the morning, set another 30-minute timer and you can put a load of laundry in the washer, empty the dishwasher, make your bed, and wipe down the kitchen counters. Before you leave the house, transfer your laundry load to the dryer. All other bigger tasks like mopping, vacuuming, and such can be put on your Task List or schedule depending on your activities and time.

Don't feel like you have to get everything done every day. Giving yourself 30 minutes of focused effort on smaller tasks will relieve stress and help you gain some control without becoming overwhelmed. Wouldn't you rather come home to a clean load of laundry every day than have mountains of dirty clothes piling up?

Stuck in Your Comfort Zone?

Most of us usually stick to our normal routines and don't like change. Because of this, we do not seek or make any changes, even though we may not be happy or satisfied with parts of our lives. Fear and anxiety about any challenge or goal will hold us back if we ask questions of ourselves like, "What if I fail?" When I started my self-improvement courses, I could no longer cling to the reasons that were holding me back and keeping, me in my comfort zone.

The comfort zone is that small area that we create with boundaries. We feel safe there and don't take risks. Many think that this is the best they can do without letting themselves grow or accept a personal or professional challenge. For example, if you are a doctor and are comfortable with the daily routines in your clinic, this is your comfort zone. You may be nervous to record a video and upload it online to give people more information about their health, even though you have great information that might improve others' lives. Making videos or public speaking is outside of your comfort zone.

Our comfort zone holds us back from massive happiness and success. I lived in my comfort zone for years. Like many women, all I wanted was to have children and raise them, which I still think is one of the greatest roles anyone can play in life. As soon I realized that I would have a harder road of infertility, I had to get out of my comfort zone, and I started to challenge my mind and body.

Getting more information about my goal was the first step. We can sometimes get nervous because we are scared to fall off course. We are learning new information and need to determine what makes sense and what doesn't and that can be scary. It is human nature to have a fear of the unknown. I educated myself to the point that when I visited a doctor's office, they thought I was educated in the medical field myself!

I got out of my comfort zone to search for someone in a similar situation who reached their goal. I emailed any women who shared their infertility story to ask them for their path to success. I paid thousands of dollars, not for treatment this time, but to get information and take online courses.

Once I got the information I needed, I put that knowledge into action. Step by step, with positive energy, I started.

Chapter 17

Persevere and Have Patience

Pursue with Perseverance

When you want to reach a goal, try to find out as much as you can about how to achieve your dream. Whether your goal is starting a business, learning a new skill, or having a baby, having facts and learning about other peoples' experience will help you.

On my journey to motherhood, I started looking for the missing information and clearing up misleading information. As a result, I came to two conclusions. First, we had already tried almost everything in the medical field in several countries. I tried medication to introduce ovulation, triggers shots, intrauterine insemination known as IUI, in vitro including egg retrieval and embryo transfer, fresh transfer, frozen transfer, 3-day embryos, 5-day embryos, and 7-day embryos. I had so many ultrasounds, hysterosalpingography x-rays, and uterine laparoscopy. The results were no pregnancy, chemical pregnancy, blighted ovum, and heartbreaking early miscarriages.

Secondly, I needed to find a new way. After my last two failed IVF procedures, I asked if there was a new protocol to try. At the time, it seemed I had already tried all that modern medicine could provide. It was up to me to figure out a new way. If you are trying to reach a goal for years, and haven't succeeded, it might be a time to consider changing your mindset and your methods. You may also want to consider asking different questions.

It is also like this with our relationships. Have you ever thought about a problem or main issue with your spouse, parents, children, or friends? Sometimes we deal with the same issue for years, but never consider changing the way we treat, talk, or behave with them, or how we react to the other person. What kind of improvement could you have in a relationship if you took a step back and didn't always engage in an argument? There are many books on improving personal relationships, so I won't go into that here, but a small change in kindness or accepting someone's personality traits can make a huge impact.

Imagine you enter a field full of rocks and someone tells you there is a hidden treasure under one of the rocks. You will probably go in all directions and lift every rock in that field to get the treasure. That is exactly what I did when I started researching the medical options for fertility treatments. I looked at alternatives and enrolled in courses to learn more. If you want to fulfill any dream, you need to make it your project to be informed. Start looking under the rocks.

I learned that if you want to achieve something, find someone who reached that goal and do what they do. For example, if you are looking for marriage advice, do not ask your divorced friend. Look for someone who has a great relationship with their spouse and get advice from them. Don't take financial advice from a friend who doesn't live within their means and is always broke. You may have people in your life who want to give you advice, but you can always listen politely and make your own decisions based on knowledge and not based on other peoples' opinions.

While on the road of pursuing your goal, do not limit yourself to imagining one specific way to achieve it. Imagine that your goal requires you to go to another state or country. Does it matter whether you get there by airplane, car, train, car, bus, or boat? In the end, the most important thing is to reach your destination. Focus on the goal and don't get bogged down in the small obstacles or hurdles. For me, I was looking only at the medical field (especially IVF) and I thought this is was the only way, and if that didn't work, nothing would work.

I opened my mind to different ways to reach my goal within my personal and religious boundaries. For us, donor egg or sperm was not an option, as it is against what we believe. For some, they might get their answers and success from medical procedures, which is fantastic! IVF or other treatments are successful for many people. I always recommend that couples seek every possible way to achieve the goal of having a baby. However, do not limit it to just medical treatment. Add a healthier lifestyle, which includes knowing what is in the foods you eat, what you drink, and beginning an exercise program. Of course, you don't have to limit yourself to these changes, but these are what helped me.

I didn't forget my mental health, either, which I think was the most important part. I listened to and watched lots of motivational speeches by famous speakers and coaches around the world. That was my first step, even when I was skeptical about doing their exercises in the beginning. But they proved me wrong. By immersing yourself in self-help videos, books, or positive messages, you will change your mindset and constantly find inspiration and new tools to help you. Surround yourself with positive examples to give you energy and motivation.

Patience

Every time I wanted something really badly, the goal moved further away from me or took longer than I wanted it to. I learned to be patient and seek my goal with a more stable emotional status. I looked at the big picture of wanting to be a mother, but I also needed to enjoy my current life while seeking my goal. Have you ever lost something and looked everywhere for it? Later on, you either quit looking or buy a new one, and you will find that lost item right in front of you. This is life! The more you want something, and the more time it takes, the more patience you will need.

It is like planting a seed in the spring. You will need to wait for summer and sometimes longer for that plant to grow and give you fruit or shade, but in the meantime, you need to take care of the plant. You need good lighting, water, good dirt, the right pot, and patience.

I treated my body as a unique plant that required different needs from a regular flower. My sister could get pregnant easily without even trying. A friend wasn't even planning on a baby and first considered her pregnancy a mistake. My neighbor got pregnant with her first IVF treatment and a colleague got pregnant using the same ovary stimulation medication that I used for over a year.

It's OK. My body is unique and I needed a little more than a pot of dirt and some water to bloom. By being patient, I could enjoy the road more to reach my dream. Patience isn't easy, and in such an emotional time as trying to get pregnant, I had sad moments and days where everything felt like a burden. But through life changes and attitude changes, I was able to persevere and stay on track to achieve my goal. Just making changes to my diet had a huge impact on my gut health and brain health. I truly feel amazing now.

Have you ever wondered why hikers spend days and nights to reach the top of the mountains? Is it fun dealing with weather changes, limited food and water, and physical exhaustion? Wouldn't it be easier for them to rent a helicopter and see the view from the top? These climbers are not just in it for the view. They enjoy the process to reach their goals, including difficulties and challenges. It takes a lot of patience to climb a mountain, and our goals sometimes seem like huge mountains.

I practice patience by slowing down and enjoying every day that Allah has gifted me. Meditation, deep breathing, positive self-talk in the mirror, and realizing my value all helped me put things into perspective and develop patience. I visualized how great it would be to be a mother. Doing these things daily helped me convince myself I would reach my goal.

I try to mention five things I am blessed with daily to give me satisfaction about my life and remind myself to be thankful. During our fourteen years of infertility, I kept telling myself that I loved my life, I had an amazing life already, and nothing was missing in my life. Adding a child to our family would make it happier and joyous, but I needed to remember the joy we already had.

There are so many people who didn't have the chance to live for today and don't have the basic needs met as most of us have. I will make my day amazing, no matter the circumstances around me. I will create my happiness from my inside. It is between my hands. I am happy with the way I am living, but I am also looking forward to making it better.

Chapter 18

Acceptance and Change

Acceptance

I never accepted that I might not have children in my life. To be more specific, I was living with resistance and rejection from within me. Working on my self-development skills, I learned that acceptance does not mean giving up. I thought that if I accepted the fact that having a baby was a dream too far out of reach then I was giving up. I will never give up on any dreams or goals I planned. For me, I consider that everything is possible to reach. I didn't accept that I wouldn't have a baby, but I did accept that it would be a difficult process. Acceptance is a peaceful psychological act that reduces stress on our bodies and minds.

Think about accepting your children the way they are. What about your spouse's annoying habit or that job you don't like anymore? Think about your relationships with family and friends. Have you tried to accept others just the way they are? We all have different beliefs, religion, and cultures. Regardless of what other people may say or do, it's most important that you accept yourself, be nice to yourself, and treat yourself nicely. You may have made huge mistakes in life, but you learned from them. We all make mistakes. You aren't going to like or support everyone's choices, but you can accept certain things, the same way that you would want others to accept you.

Stop blaming yourself for not raising your children the way you dreamed you would. There is always time to fix, create, and change. Make it a priority to change a situation you aren't happy about. A quick example is watching your husband's favorite sport on TV. You don't have to like sports or want to go to games. But you don't need to reject it and dampen his enjoyment of sports. Go with the flow and improve yourself daily.

It was hard and I needed a lot of practice to accept my infertility issues, but I did. I had an honest talk with myself—just me and myself—in my favorite place in my backyard. We talked to each other and I accepted that my body was at this stage and in this condition. I would not be able to get pregnant. I got it! I accepted that I was dealing with unexplained infertility, even though my body did have some physical issues. Frequent failed IVF attempts convinced me it was unexplained and there was something hidden that doctors were missing. I would accept my condition, "unexplained infertility," and fix it. "Unexplained" doesn't mean unknowable. We just didn't have an answer…yet. Then I asked myself, *What steps should I do to improve my health and my body to a phase that it is ready to get pregnant naturally?*

Change

"Healthy lifestyle" is a very broad subject, but I chose to focus on three points and began implementing new habits in three categories: healthy eating, physical exercise, and mental health.

I switched to clean eating and healthy food as much as possible. I started researching dietary changes that boost infertility, such as gluten-free products, organic products, and, as much as I could, I limited sugar and processed food. I also went off of caffeine and drank a lot of water.

Depending on your condition, there are many dietary changes you can make to improve your health.

I began exercising every day at the same time. I found certain exercises that were known to help with infertility. I'm not giving medical advice or making any claims, just letting you know what worked for me. I focused on exercises that that targeted belly fat, walked a lot, and started practicing infertility yoga. For 40 minutes every day, I would rotate between my exercises and end it with my favorite yoga poses. Daily exercise helps to manage stress.

Breathing exercises are essential for stress management. Every morning before I started my day, I would take ten deep breaths. As I did this, I would remind myself of four amazing things in my life that I am grateful for:

1. My health. Even with the infertility problems, I can walk, hear, see, and enjoy life.
2. My family. I can see my family every day and receive the love and support they provide and do the same for them.
3. My husband. I have the most supportive and caring husband in this world. We have misunderstandings and disagreements, like any couple. We faced hard times, especially related to infertility, but we still managed to improve our marriage and continue to grow together.
4. Our financial life. We have food to eat, a house to live in, and a car to take us where we need to go. These basic things are a dream for millions of people around the world.

I started to realize how grateful I was! That gratitude helped me focus on the positive areas in my life. I opened my eyes to see even more blessings and appreciate flowers, trees, sun, moon, neighbors, and every little thing that I didn't see or feel before.

Accepting myself and my situation helped me love my life and gave me more time to enjoy things instead of complaining or crying when I needed to. Sometimes we all need to get something off our chest, but we can still appreciate what we have.

I became more aware of my mental health needs. I learned that it is OK *not* to be OK for an hour or so, but also I learned to get these negative feelings out through crying, especially hard sobbing for ten minutes. Letting yourself cry for a bit helps your whole body get out all that negative energy that has built up inside you for years. You may have been trying to prove you are strong, but after that ten minutes, you can dry your eyes and move forward. Once you do this, you can face essential life challenges that help you to become stronger and prepared for success. You will even notice that you don't need to complain because you learned to accept something and didn't let that negative energy take over.

Before working in American society and familiarizing myself with a new culture, I thought that only my Middle Eastern people cared so much about having babies. It was a frequent topic of conversation. But this seems to be universal. Everyone asks new couples when they are going to start having children. It must be human nature.

In my culture, especially in my small village in Palestine, having children is very valued. After getting married, within months people will start asking if you are excepting. I wished I could say "yes," but while dealing with infertility for over 14 years, I kept explaining why we didn't have children. This was so hard for me and I ended up crying when one of these random people, family, or friends would give us advice or recommend a doctor. The worst was when someone would say, "I feel sorry for you guys."

After I invested in myself and improved my coping skills and my attitude, I changed that feeling to positive energy. Every time someone mentioned babies, medical advice, or gave me sympathy, I told myself how nice these people were, how beloved and lucky I was to have them around! I focused on how thoughtful they were to share their experience with me. Accepting their questions as concern, and not judgment, helped a lot. Switching and changing that feeling was a blessing that I gifted to myself.

Chapter 19

Failure and Forgiveness

Failure

Be prepared to fail before you reach your goal. Failure can teach us more than anything else. It provides a challenge to make our goal even more special and lets us see obstacles we didn't expect. If you reach success in one area easily, that is awesome! In general, failure is predictable. However, it will show you the strength you have and challenge you to find another way to move forward.

Do you remember your first steps in life? Probably not, but I know your parents remember. How many times did you fall before you succeeded? You needed practice and support from your parents to learn that amazing skill and now you don't even notice that your body is doing something huge when you are walking. You took years to learn words, put sentences together, and to read. Now you speak with ease, flow, and confidence. You probably don't even think twice about the practice and learning it took for you to read this book right now. These skills required a lot of failure and practice to achieve and they are small miracles that you should be grateful for.

When I was trying to get pregnant, every failed treatment broke me down because of the high expectations I created in my mind. Chances are not high with every cycle of IVF, but still, I thought I was making such a huge effort that should pay off. But I learned that after all those failed attempts, there was a huge success hidden behind it, and I was right. Natural pregnancy with twins was a great accomplishment that Allah rewarded me with after all of the failure. When I accepted failure, I chose to improve my chances in another way by working on myself.

Did I learn from those failures? Of course! There is nothing in my life that taught me like my failure. Failure taught me patience, pain, hope, and helped me see the value and worth of life, family, friends, and my child. Having Rawhi has brought a big responsibility on my shoulders to educate myself and try my best to raise and teach him to be a good person in this world.

Never let your dream fly away from you. You can do it. If others can reach their goals, you can, too. Motivate yourself because no one will motivate you. Help yourself, because you can't expect others to have all the answers. Get up, set a goal, plan to achieve it, and do the work. Start enjoying the challenge, learn from failures, and keep moving forward. No matter what others say about your dream, keep going. I stopped talking about my dream and kept it to myself. Not because I was weak, but because I wanted to quit being impacted by negative people around me. This made me feel stronger.

Forgiveness

While pursuing your dreams, do yourself a favor and forgive. Forgiveness is a gift for our heart that will help you reach a peaceful level of living. Forgive yourself about silly and stupid mistakes you did. You are human, and all humans make mistakes. Forgive your family, spouse, children, friends, or anyone that you have some resentment about. Forgiveness is not easy, but you can do it for yourself. That doesn't mean you need to stay in an abusive situation or accept bad behavior. You can still move on from the person who is hurting you.

There are several practices I did to learn to forgive. I put myself in the other person's shoes and tried to understand their actions. I also remembered times when I made a mistake and made someone feel bad. That person forgave me, so I needed to forgive others, too.

I looked in the mirror and imagined I was talking to them to get out everything I was feeling in my heart. I screamed at their image that I pictured in the mirror. I told them that they hurt me, but I also told them, *I forgive you because I am strong with a big heart and am not letting anyone hurt me.* Forgiveness doesn't always mean telling them in person that you forgive them, especially if they don't accept that they have hurt you.

If all these recommendations do not work, talk to a therapist. A professional can help you understand your situation, guide you as you work through those feelings, and help you see a way to forgive. You don't have to stay in a bad relationship or accept others hurting you. Forgiveness is for your heart and is a way of moving on.

Chapter 20

Believe and Have Faith

Believe

Believe in your dream, live it, talk about it to yourself, and visualize your goal as if it is already achieved. Close your eyes and create a mental image with all the details and include your senses to help see your goal and live it completely Do this a couple of times a day. Imagine your dream or you might write it down on a big piece of paper. Imagine yourself moving toward your dream, passing all the challenges and steps required.

Is your goal to start your own business? Use your imagination to create a visual picture of that business. What kind of business is it? Do you have a building? If so, picture what it would look like. How many people are working with you? Picture yourself having more time and money to travel because of your new business. Think of the new house you will buy and how you can build your own house, increase your wealth, and help others.

Then get up and start working. Imagination alone will not help you reach your goal. It is a great motivational tool, but it should be associated with real steps and work. Making this goal real in your mind will provide you with motivation and get your brain to work faster. In other words, this kind of focused visualization decreases the amount of time needed to reach your goals.

Every day I imagined how I would feel when I found out that I was pregnant. I pictured the way I would tell my husband and announce my pregnancy. I lived in my imagination, created those feelings associated with it, and kept working. If you trick your brain with your dream, your brain will work harder to achieve it. Our brains are complex and can be trained to accept imagination as truth. In this stage, I lived the dream completely and treated myself as a pregnant woman. It may sound strange, but by visualizing my pregnancy, I was helping my brain and body reach the goal.

Faith

Faith is a central part of my life. Walking in the early morning gave me such a gift as I looked around and saw all of Allah's amazing creations. My faith increased as I associated gratitude for Allah in my prayers. I grew up in a Muslim family and I consider myself a good Muslim, but as a human, I do make mistakes and I ask Allah for forgiveness.

Through the years, I was saying that I was thankful to Allah, no matter what. But to be honest, I think I wasn't really feeling thankful. Deep inside, I was yelling, "Why me?" Now, I get it and I ask Allah to forgive me for my doubts. Why me? Why not me? In the holy Quran, Allah says in Sura Ghafir 60, "Call upon me, I will respond to you," but I was asking Allah for years why I didn't get my answer when I wanted it.

I realized that maybe I needed to change my ways. I started to make *duaa* (prayer) with certainty that my prayer would be answered, and I finished my prayer with a big smile. He is my God and He is the most powerful. He will lead me to a way to reach my dream and He did. Making *duaa* daily was like therapy for my tired soul. I told Allah I was doing the best I could and had faith He would answer my prayer. I started to feel so much better and refreshed as soon as I finished my *duaa*.

The faith that increased in my heart improved my overall physical and mental health. I started to glow more! Family and friends asked what I was doing. They could see a visible change in my appearance and spirit. I started to look for other ways to bring happiness to my heart. What else could I do to make myself happy? They say if you make someone else happy, you will get twice the happiness. I decided to try it.

I started to look for ways to make others happy in my community, school, family, and anyone in need. Every day I drew a smile on my face. I said, "Good Morning" with a big smile to my neighbors. I would get my friend her favorite drink without her asking for it. I told my mom that I missed her. I did small things like sending my husband a love message and telling my sister she looks beautiful. These are small ways to spread happiness. Kindness is free. I also looked for bigger ways to help others, like volunteering with children and the homeless. There are so many ways to create happiness within yourself by creating it for others. Did I get twice the happiness? NO! I got much more than that.

Down deep in our hearts we love helping others. Sometimes we don't think we can help others because of financial issues and lack of time. Providing money or time to a charity makes a difference in the community. Donating money, things, or time, such as volunteering, will raise your self-esteem and your feeling of value and worth in this life. You will meet new people who share the same interests and passions. More relationships means more opportunities to succeed in life.

Meeting new people could help in any area of your life. Imagine that you have an online business selling goods. Knowing new people means potential new customers, which will be beneficial to you. You may be able to connect a new realtor acquaintance with a friend who is selling their house. Donating to charity feels good. Have you ever tried to take gifts and visit a nursing home, orphanage, or anyone in need in your family or community?

I divide every paycheck into three categories. First are basic life expenses such as bills, mortgage, utilities, and food. Second, I put a percentage of every check in savings. That percentage will change based on your expenses or budget. Third is a percentage that goes to charity. I set a date in my calendar every month that I must donate an amount of money to charity. This has really made me a happier person.

One of my favorite charity ideas that brings joy to me is creating and donating hospital bags for women in need in other countries. These bags include everything they will need to take with them to the hospital to deliver their babies. I still smile as I think of the baby clothes and new mommy essentials I packed for myself before delivering my own babies. Doing this for other new moms helps me "pay it forward" and pass on that gratitude. The great feeling I receive is Allah's reward to me for giving and thinking of others' needs.

Chapter 21

Reward and Appreciation

Reward Yourself

No matter what you are going through, you are worthy! You are valued and you need to appreciate yourself because if you don't do it now, no one else will. Never allow anyone to bully you, make you feel small, or be a victim to the acts or words of another person. You are a human and you do make a difference in this world.

Take a moment and think about all you have accomplished and your roles in life. Are you a wife, mother, daughter, husband, father, student, employee, or business owner? What is your role? You will probably count five roles in which you have succeeded and feel valued. Take time to appreciate yourself and reward yourself for every goal or achievement you meet.

Get yourself a good gift, wrap it the way you like, and enjoy it. I finished my bachelor's and master's degrees through an online university. Every time I finished a course, I would reward myself with something simple like an ice cream cup at the drive-thru or a new book to read.

Even though I buy a lot of books, I made sure to consider that book a special reward. After every term I finished, I rewarded myself with a better gift, like a new pair of sneakers or an online course about self-development skills. For my big goals and achievements, I rewarded myself with a vacation. No matter your income, you can give yourself a reward that will make you happy, even if it is small.

Look at yourself in the mirror and talk to yourself about how much you appreciate yourself, your kindness to others, your financial support, and the love and care you provide. You are complete. You don't need others' approval to tell you how beautiful you are from inside and out.

Be kind to yourself and avoid self-criticism. If you made a big mistake toward someone or yourself, just apologize and remind yourself to avoid repeating it in the future. Allow others to compliment you. If you are wearing a nice dress and someone says it a beautiful dress, just say "Thank you." Every time I wear something new, I patiently wait for my husband to give me a compliment, but this is not always the case. It would be nice, but I know I look good no matter what.

Most men will never notice your new lipstick color or new hairstyle, because their thinking is different than ours. Women tend to see details and notice changes more than men do. After I worked on myself and appreciated myself more, I stopped waiting for him to compliment my new outfit, hair, or makeup because I already knew I looked my best. To my surprise, he started to notice more, and I started to get more compliments. I just smiled and said, "Thank you!"

Appreciation

Appreciate your body. If you are reading this, I guarantee your heart is beating, you are breathing, and your brain is thinking. Walking, eating, and moving our bodies are gifts that we don't even notice. Thank your body and appreciate it.

I found fasting a couple of days a month helped cleanse my body and strengthen its systems. As a Muslim, we have Ramadan, which is a whole month of fasting from sunrise to sunset. It helps clean your body and spirit and get ready for another eleven months. In addition to Ramadan, I did this a few days a month and my body loved it. I will not eat food or drink from sunrise to sunset, then break my fast with a light soup. Then I prepare a delicious meal, such as roasted chicken with vegetables, with a healthy salad on the side. I also drank a lot of water to clean my body from all unhealthy food and give my cells more hydration.

I also began treating my body better by eating living food. Living food is any food that will grow if you take it and plant it in your garden. Vegetables, fruits, and legumes are all living food. I stayed away from any food that goes through machines or is processed. I avoided them completely. Within three weeks, my skin started to glow, my energy level increased, and my overall health improved. I thought I was appreciating my body by working hard in other ways, but eating better made a huge difference.

Start appreciating your surroundings. I started to see things I never paid attention to before. I will thank Allah for that every day. I live in Chicago, and winter weather is not the best for most people, but I love everything. I never complain about snow, heat, humidity, or rainy days. Look for the everyday beauty of life.

I also began appreciating the time I could spend outside. I aimed for 30 minutes a day outside in the sun to get vitamin D as much as I could. When I was tested, it was discovered that I had a vitamin D deficiency. Does it have an impact to my infertility? I don't know about that, but it definitely impacts my overall health. Searching for a good supplement to take daily was a chore. Chicago weather has long winters and very humid summers and it is difficult to get all of my vitamin D just from the sun. I was able to take one multivitamin that supported my body with needed supplements. I took it daily before bedtime.

Walking barefoot for half an hour a day during my sun time outside had great benefits. Connecting to Mother Earth with no boundaries helps to increase your body's overall health. It may sound weird, but there is a connection between your body and the earth. There are electrons that can reduce inflammation that we receive and feel through our skin by connecting with the earth. It was a new experience for me, and it helped me to feel that connection while walking outside the house barefoot. My best experience of feeling that connection was while walking on the beach when we were in Cancun, Mexico.

We delayed our honeymoon for financial reasons, but finally decided to visit Cancun after we had been married for twelve years. This was strictly a honeymoon. No doctors, no clinics. We made an agreement that we would not talk about our infertility or mention anything about it for the whole week.

We spoiled ourselves with a beautiful hotel suite and we celebrated ourselves and our many years of marriage. It was one of the most amazing trips we went on. Meditation, yoga, and walking barefoot during sunrise were incredible experiences. The resort was adults only, which helped a lot with keeping the agreement we made. We totally forgot about kids and infertility and had a special time. I still remember and feel every moment.

Chapter 22

Expectations and Reasons

Expectations

If you look back on the bigger disappointments in your life, do you notice that some of them came from the higher expectations you built up in your head? That's exactly what happened to me. With every IVF treatment, I had very high expectations, of course, because of our relatively good health and because it was a known successful treatment. I thought my optimism was called "positive energy," but in fact, it was high expectations.

It is the same thing in our relationships with others. When we expect something specific from others and they do not provide it, we feel sad and heartbroken. We expect our partners to take care of us if we are sick, and if they don't provide support, we feel miserable and blame them for not loving us as much as we love them.

When someone fails to meet our expectations, we sometimes ignore the fact that they might have had a tough day (worse than ours), they may be sick, or they just didn't notice or thought we didn't need anything.

Love shows itself in many different ways and, after years, it is still love, but may take a different shape. Men generally show love through actions such as providing support, safety, and taking care of the children. They don't always think of the smaller ways they can show love. This is a time to lower your expectations and appreciate what you have.

We expect our children to get great grades in school and behave properly, but when they don't, we feel anxious and blame ourselves for not raising them right. At every parent-teacher conference we had at our school, there were some parents who left sad and angry. Their child's performance didn't match their high expectations. Parents sometimes ignore the fact that they need to be closer to their kids, figure out their personalities and abilities, and help and support them in any way they can.

I understand that we all want our children to be the best in every area, not just school, but honestly, every child is unique. Learning methods and ways to motivate each child is important. Not all plants will grow strong and bloom in the same soil, water, and sunlight.

Don't wait for anything from anyone. In other words, do not expect. Take expectation out of your life. Your good deeds are rewarded by Allah, so do not wait for anything from anyone. If someone provides you with something, that's great! If not, don't take it personally. If you love compliments, give them to yourself. Look in the mirror and say, "What a beautiful dress! I look gorgeous!"

Motivate yourself and protect yourself from negative thoughts or negative people around you. Sometimes it is tough, because the one who tries to put you down could be someone who is very close to you. Take a step back or face them. This is one of the best things I've learned and put into practice.

Let's say I am trying to reach my goal and someone is trying to hold me back or put me down. I do one of the two practices. I will talk to them and ask why they are putting me down. I try to understand their point of view. Maybe they have their experience to share; good or bad.

The second thing I do is avoid talking about my dream with that person. I can still have a good relationship with them, and we can talk about other things, but I know this issue will only get a negative response from them. I look for people who are sharing the same dream. I joined private groups through social media filled with people around the world who were also dealing with infertility. Those people have experience, inspiration, and we share motivation and encouragement with each other.

When watching a great movie, we only see what is onscreen. We don't see behind the scenes and learn the problems they faced to reach the goal of creating this perfect movie. Was one of the actors a brat on set? Did the money run out or go over budget? These are the things we don't consider when enjoying a movie. This is exactly how our lives unfold. We don't see the things that are happening behind the scenes.

Reasons

Everything happens for a reason. People say this a lot, but sometimes you won't see the bigger picture until you are out of a bad situation or reach that goal. Do you remember when a relationship didn't work out with a person and you were left heartbroken? Afterward, you met another amazing person who deserves your care and love. Do you remember feeling broken because your business failed or you didn't get the job you wanted? Now you have a better career and are in a better financial situation. Life is a series of stations that we stop at to reach our final destination.

You can picture these as train stations or rest stops along the highway on a long trip. Some are clean and pleasant and others are scary and messy. If you have ever been to a dirty bathroom in a gas station, you can picture exactly what I am describing! In the end, you don't give it a lot of thought if you realize that you are just passing through to reach your final destination. Be flexible. We want to reach our goal, but it doesn't matter what road we are taking. If one road is under construction, you may need to take a detour. It's is like this in life. If you only seek perfection in life and want everything to happen according to your plans, you will be disappointed easily.

No matter the path, just keep moving forward. Your life is valuable and your time is important. Learn more about your goal, read and educate yourself, and build new habits to keep you focused on your own life. Don't get bogged down in other peoples' drama. When I finished my associate's degree, I wanted to enroll and finish my bachelor's degree right away. However, college tuition was very high so I could not continue at that time. I started selling products online through e-commerce websites to save for my tuition.

Because of this detour, I finished my bachelor's degree and wanted to seek my master's. At that time, the only job I found was as a teacher's assistant in addition to my online shop. I took that job to reach my dream and achieved the goal of getting my master's degree. I love education, but being a full-time teacher was not my dream for my whole life. It was a station in my life and I loved it.

I love having flexibility in life and I didn't see myself working in a traditional job from eight to four every day. However, I was flexible and took the job as a station on the way to my larger goal of starting a family. Start seeking your dream but keep something on the side to provide you with income to live and survive. While doing that work on your big dream, you will be amazed at how life will reward you.

Nine IVF treatments failed for reasons that I didn't understand at that time. Despite the failures, it taught me to take care of myself, develop new skills, and be the person I am now. I imagine if I got pregnant and had children right after marriage, I don't think I would be in the stage I am in right now.

Failure will show you these reasons. It taught me how to be successful, helped me seek different ways, and ultimately, I reached my dream. Failure created a stronger relationship between my husband and me because we lived through the suffering together. Failure taught me how to be creative, believe, and achieve.

Chapter 23

Find Happiness

Look for happiness everywhere every day and add it to your life. Rawhi survived, made it home, and we couldn't be happier. As I write this, he still has an NG tube for feeding, but it is just a station for him. He is eight months old, well-adjusted, and hearing his sweet laughter throughout the house is worth every moment of waiting to have him.

I still do things that make myself happy. Now when I look in the mirror, it is not just me. I hold my son and tell myself how amazing we are together. I tell him how much I love him every day, all the time. Saying "I love you," has a great impact in my heart, too.

Take a couple of moments and think about what really makes you happy. If you didn't find a quick answer, start to explore your life and write down some positive things. You might be surprised that a little thing like saying "hi" to others, more "thank you" and "please," or feeding the birds brings a lot of joy to your tired heart. Happiness is indeed a decision and, no matter what, we need to decide to be happy. Flipping negative things around and looking for the positive side will help you stay at your Royal Stage. I call this a Royal Stage because you will be living in your own luxury inside a peaceful world that will start to show in your glowing face. You will feel like a queen.

Looking for win-win situations is a rule that you should follow in your life. As soon as you start to love yourself, which is not the same as being selfish, you will be amazed at the love other people will show you. We sometimes mistake self-love with selfishness, but there is a huge difference. Self-love is taking care of yourself. Buy something new for yourself, improve your education without needing others to motivate you. Be generous to yourself and don't criticize yourself. You deserve it.

Self-love is seeking happiness and love for myself in order to provide it to others, such as my spouse, my family members, my community, and everyone around me. Being selfish is hard work with negative connotation. Selfish people see only themselves in the world and their priority is only their own needs or own successes. They don't care about others and it shows in the way that they treat people.

One part of selfishness is jealousy. Stop comparing yourself to others. It is one of the worst ways to destroy ourselves inside and, ultimately, destroy your happiness. Not everything we see is true, especially on social media. If you could see what other peoples' problems are, you would probably be glad you don't have their life, even if they come across as perfect and beautiful. Instead, look at someone as a good example or what they have as something to aspire to and don't let jealousy kill your spirit.

Choose your path in life. Be creative, colorful, and unique. Be a good listener and avoid unnecessary discussions where you want to express your own opinion to someone who won't change their mind. Pass on relationships that take too much effort (and emotion). Concentrate instead on positive relationships and happy people.

Once you reach this Royal Stage, be prepared for success in everything you do! Every goal is attainable and you have the power and the tools to reach it. Achieving success and reaching your goals becomes a habit. Once your reach one goal, the things you learned and the successes and failures you experienced along the way will help you reach other goals. You are now building on your pattern of achievement and putting those lessons you learned into practice. You are creating happiness.

Final Thoughts

I learned to understand what my body needed for a successful pregnancy and it became a roadmap for success. Today I am twenty weeks pregnant with my third baby naturally, without spending years of my life to achieve it. This is the first time I experienced a surprise pregnancy. I wasn't really planning for it. I wanted to give Rawhi time to grow stronger and bigger, especially with his specific needs that come with being a premature baby with delayed milestones and a long list of therapies and appointments. To be honest, it was one of the most special and happy surprises I received in my life. It is a blessing that Allah rewarded me for the struggle and hard time I had after losing Yaseen. Rawhi will have the chance to grow up close in age with his brother or sister! Won't that be amazing?

We don't need to go through our own hardships to learn. We need to learn from others' experiences and advice. For example, it took me 14 years to achieve my goal and now I am putting everything I learned in this book to help others achieve their goal in a shorter period of time.

Fourteen years and I tried not to give up, but I did. Then I made changes to my life, raised my head up, and kept walking and moving toward my goals. I learned the secrets that make any dream reachable in a shorter amount of time. At the beginning of this book I called myself a wife, daughter, elementary school educator, fertility warrior, and an author. I've achieved my lifelong goal and now I cherish my favorite title of all: Mama.

I hope that by sharing my experiences, lessons, and knowledge, I have encouraged you and given you hope to pursue your dreams and goals, too. This is my own personal story. No extra dramatic events were added and, as you read, you can see I didn't need any extra drama. Stories are another person's life given to us to learn from. I want you to stay motivated, stay strong, and know that you are a valuable human being. You can achieve your dreams.

Once you have reached your goal, I would love to hear from you! I want to support you and celebrate with you. I look forward to your feedback, thoughts, and experiences. My goal seemed very natural and easy for most people, but for me, it took me what seemed like a lifetime to reach it. No matter what your goal is, make it big, worthy, and something that adds value to your life. Enjoy the journey, be patient, and remember that your experiences are just a station on the long road of life. Along the way, spread kindness to others, appreciate your surroundings, and let it go. Forgive others and live your life peacefully.

With my love, support, and prayers,
Neveen Musa
Neveenmusa56@gmail.com

Made in the USA
Monee, IL
27 September 2020